Medical Law, Ethics, and Bioethics for Ambulatory Care

Fourth Edition

Medical Law, Ethics, and Bioethics for Ambulatory Care

Fourth Edition

MARCIA (MARTI) A. LEWIS, EdD, RN, CMA-AC
Associate Dean, Mathematics, Science and Health Occupations

Instructor, Medical Assisting
Olympic College
Bremerton, Washington

CAROL D. TAMPARO, PhD, CMA-A
Dean, Business and Allied Health
Lake Washington Technical College
Kirkland, Washington

 F. A. DAVIS COMPANY • **Philadelphia**

F. A. Davis Company
1915 Arch Street
Philadelphia, PA 19103

Printed in the United States of America

Last digit indicates print number: 10 9 8 7 6 5 4 3 2 1

Publisher, Health Professions: Jean-François Vilain
Developmental Editor: Marianne Fithian
Cover Design by: Louis J. Forgione

Library of Congress Cataloging-in-Publication Data

Lewis, Marcia A.
    Medical law, ethics, and bioethics for ambulatory care / Marcia (Marti) A. Lewis,
Carol D. Tamparo.—4th ed.
        p. cm.
    Rev. ed. of: Medical law, ethics, and bioethics in the medical office / Marcia (Marti) A.
Lewis, Carol D. Tamparo. 3rd ed. c1993.
    Includes bibliographical references and index.
    ISBN 0-8036-0348-7
    1. Medical laws and legislation—United States.   2. Medical ethics—United States.
3. Ambulatory medical care—Law and legislation—United States. I. Tamparo,
Carol D., 1940–   .
II. Lewis, Marcia A. Medical law, ethics, and bioethics in the medical office. III. Title.
KF3821.L485   1998
344.73'041—dc21   97-50565
                                                                                                          CIP

Preface

It is imperative that the ambulatory care employee have a knowledge of medical law, ethics, and bioethics so that the client may be treated with understanding, sensitivity, and compassion. No matter what the employee's education and experience, any direct client contact involves ethical and legal responsibility. It also is imperative that this knowledge be used to provide the best possible service for the physician employer. Our goal is to provide the employee with an adequate resource for the study of medical law, ethics, and bioethics.

Although the material is applicable to all health care professionals in any setting, our emphasis continues to be on the ambulatory health care setting rather than the hospital or long-term care setting. For example, we do not address such legal and bioethical issues as whether or not to feed an anencephalic newborn in the neonatal center of the hospital because this book's focus is on the ambulatory health care setting. We realize, however, that all bioethical issues may affect ambulatory health care personnel. Enthusiastic feedback from instructors, students, and reviewers is gratifying and has resulted in many changes that will make this fourth edition an even more useful resource than the first three editions. We are reminded of the truth, which comes from colleagues in our respective community and technical colleges, that no matter how many times a piece is written, it can always be improved.

This revision is necessitated by the continuing evolution of health care, of legal and, especially, bioethical issues. The material is updated throughout the book to reflect the latest developments. The new title more accurately reflects the growing ambulatory health care setting. The material in the law chapters is reorganized to make the progression more logical and pedagogically effective. The material in the bioethical section of the book is updated to reflect emerging ethical issues. A new chapter introducing the reader to the cultural perspectives of health care heightens our awareness of the importance of culture in health care.

The authors and their editors have made every attempt to ensure currency and pertinence of the material. However, some bioethical issues change almost daily as lawmakers and the public become actively involved and press for legislation. Managed care, physician-assisted suicide, and issues involving gene manipulation and therapy are emerging continually and are addressed in the text.

For ease of reference, the various codes of ethics appear in Appendix I. Appendix II offers samples of some of the legal documents clients may use in implementing decisions about health care, life, and death.

Reader response to the vignettes in the first three editions of the book has been remarkable. For that reason, we have added several to this edition. Some of the vignettes are adapted from actual case law, and for these we have provided the relevant citations. Other vignettes recount actual situations of which we are aware. All will whet the appetite, stimulate discussion, and highlight the most pressing legal, ethical, and bioethical issues faced by ambulatory care employees.

Each chapter is preceded by learning objectives designed for the educational setting. The discussion questions are intended to be thought provoking rather than a test of chapter contents. References are provided for anyone seeking additional information. We have included more reader-friendly life situations for discussion and application of your state statutes. We have added more case law examples to provide for further discussion.

We hope that you will derive from this book a great sense of pride for your professional position as an ambulatory health care employee.

MAL
CDT

Acknowledgments

It is never possible to acknowledge all persons who make contributions to the writers of a book. Completing a book requires assistance from too many individuals and sources. We wish to thank, however, a few who were especially helpful. Without them, the book would have been impossible. Our gratitude goes to our reviewers; their meticulous work, diligence, and commitment to medical law, ethics, and bioethics is obvious and appreciated:

Cindy A. Abel, CMA, PBT(ASCP)BS, Medical Assistant Program Chair, Department of Medical Assisting, Ivy Tech State College, Lafayette, Indiana

Bonnie L. Deister, MS, BSN, CMA-C, Assistant Professor, Chairperson, Medical Assisting/Paramedic Program, Broome Community College, Binghamton, New York

Deborah S. Gilbert, RRA, Assistant Professor, Technical Department (Medical Secretary), Dalton College, Dalton, Georgia

Rhonda K. Myers, RMA, Medical Instructor, Department of Medical Assisting, Metro Business College, Jefferson City, Missouri

Jean-François Vilain, Publisher, Health Professions, and Marianne Fithian, Developmental Editor, F. A. Davis Company, continually encouraged us throughout the writing of the fourth edition. We appreciate their ability to assist us and, when necessary, to be critical of us but with a sense of humor. Our appreciation also goes to Herbert J. Powell, Jr., Director of Editing, Design, and Production, and Carol O'Connell of Graphic World Publishing Services for assistance during the production cycle. Students in our classes continually offered current critical thought and information on legal, ethical, and bioethical issues and acted as a sounding board for all ideas. Their input and comments have influenced this product. Students continue to be our inspiration and the reason for this book!

The support of families and friends was an essential ingredient from the inception of the first edition of the book to the completion of this fourth edition. Thanks to Les and Martiann Lewis, Jayne Bloomberg and Duuana Otey, and Tom Tamparo. They relinquished their time with us so we could write. They provided encouragement when we were discouraged, and celebrated with us when we were successful. Thanks, we do love you! Last, but most important: Thanks Marti! Thanks Carol!

MAL
CDT

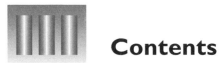

Contents

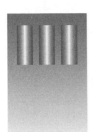

Vignettes

The vignettes are either true events or based, in part, on case law. In the former, names are changed, as are some events, to ensure clients' right to privacy. In case law, either the case law is quoted directly or it is noted as changed in part to allow the case to be more relevant to medical assistants and to the ambulatory health care setting.

Vignette I

A certified medical assistant (CMA) employed by an obstetrician/gynecologist calls her former medical assistant instructor to inform her of an opening for a clinical assistant in the obstetrics and gynecology (OB/GYN) clinic. After describing the position and its responsibilities, the CMA says, "We really need another person in the clinical area. I'm the doctor's only nurse."

Surprised by the comment, the instructor inquires, "When did you go back to school to become a nurse?"

She replies, "Oh, I didn't, but everyone thinks I am his nurse. I do everything a nurse does."

Vignette 2

As a medical assistant educator with several years of experience in the administrative area and a recognized authority on medical records, you have been asked to testify as an expert witness regarding protocol for making corrections in a medical record. You agree.

When you are interviewed by the attorney and given the records to review, you recognize that the person responsible for the data entered in the record is a former student and a practicing certified medical assistant. It appears obvious that the records have been altered after the fact.

Vignette 3

A patient seriously injures his thumb and hand on the job. A local physician cleanses and bandages the wound and administers an antitetanus injection. The doctor prescribes antibiotics and pain medication.

The patient is seen by the physician's employee for the next four visits. The medical office employee is a high school graduate who worked approximately 2 years as a nurse's aide in the local hospital before working for this doctor.

On subsequent visits, the employee removes dead tissue and cleanses and bandages the wound. The patient complains of severe pain. The employee expresses pus from the wound on several occasions. The thumb and hand become inflamed, and the patient loses range of motion.

The patient sees the doctor or his employee for 17 more visits during a 2-month period. The employee treats the patient for 12 of the 17 visits.

The patient loses full function of his hand and seeks consultation from another physician. *Delaney v Rosenthall,* 196 NE2d 878 (1966).

Vignette 4

Mrs. Farley had a tubal ligation. She was informed of the risks and signed consent forms before surgery. Five months later she returned to the same physician, who determined that she was pregnant. After the birth of Mrs. Farley's baby, the attending physician examined both of her fallopian tubes and found that one was ligated, but the other appeared normal. Mrs. Farley sued the physician who performed the tubal ligation on the basis of *res ipsa loquitur*.

Outcome: The court held that Mrs. Farley could not rely on the doctrine of *res ipsa loquitur* to establish the medical malpractice claim against the physician. The court held that "the doctrine of *res ipsa loquitur* cannot be invoked where the existence of negligence is wholly a matter of conjecture and the circumstances are not proved, but must themselves be presumed, or when it may be inferred that there was no negligence on the part of the defendant." The doctrine only holds in cases in which the defendant's negligence is the only inference that can reasonably and legitimately be drawn from the circumstances. This was not the case here. The court stated that this was probably one of those cases in which the sterilization procedure failed; the ligation was performed, but the ligation band came off soon thereafter. *Farley v Meadows*, 404 SE2d 537 (1991).

Vignette 5

Kelly, a first-year medical assistant student, tells her instructor that she thinks she may be pregnant and wonders what she should do. The instructor recommends that Kelly go to the campus health center for a pregnancy test. When Kelly's test is positive, she again discusses her case with her instructor. As a single woman, Kelly decides she cannot support a child now but is not sure whether to have the baby and put it up for adoption or to have an abortion. After a few days and a discussion with the father of the child, their decision is to have an abortion.

Kelly returns to the campus health clinic for her test results so that she can take them to the abortion clinic. The certified medical assistant, a former graduate of the school's medical assistant program and a health center employee, refuses to give Kelly the test results, saying "You'll have to talk to the nurse practitioner. I don't believe in abortion." The nurse practitioner gives her the laboratory results.

3

Vignette 6

To continue with the dilemma of Kelly's pregnancy (Vignette 5), consider the following information.

Several days later in the medical assistant clinical class, another medical assistant instructor overhears Nancy, a student who was receiving work experience in the campus health center, breach a confidence and tell other students in the class about Kelly's pregnancy and abortion.

The program's coordinator privately speaks with Nancy about the breach of confidentiality. Nancy responds, "I didn't tell the whole class. I only told my friend."

Vignette 7

A patient underwent elective surgery for total hip replacement. Early during the surgery, the assistant surgeon became so ill he had to lie down on the operating room floor. The hospital called another physician (Dr. Howard), who had his office across the street from the hospital. He canceled his office appointments, came to the hospital, and completed the surgery with the surgeon. After the surgery, the patient suffered complications and sued Dr. Howard.

Outcome: Under the Good Samaritan Law in California, the court ruled that Dr. Howard "did not commit any willful act or omission" while assisting the surgeon. Dr. Howard was rendering emergency care in "good faith," which addresses the quality of the intentions and not the quality of the care delivered. Also, Dr. Howard had no preexisting duty of professional care to this patient; the patient was not an established patient of his. This is another requirement of the Good Samaritan Law. Further, the court stated that, as a matter of public policy, the Good Samaritan Law encourages physicians to respond to emergency requests. *Perkins v Howard,* 283 Cal Rptr 764 (1991).

Note: Although this case involves physicians working in a hospital, the legal implications are strong for office assistants and office settings as well.

Vignette 8

Dr. Enke's laboratory technician explains any necessary tests to her clients as a standard procedure. The client, Smoger, was unhappy and thought he would have had much less trouble with his laboratory test had the doctor herself made the explanation.

Outcome: A federal court ruled that a doctor can have a laboratory technician tell a patient about the risks involved in a test, stating, "It violates no requirement of the law for the doctor to delegate the duty to inform."

Note: This vignette is based, in part, on *Smoger v Enke*, 874 F2d 295 (5th Cir 1989).

Vignette 9

Two gay men in their 50s desire to adopt a child. One of the men has juvenile onset diabetes and is partially blind. These partners have sufficient financial resources. They are willing to accept a child with special needs.

Vignette 10

Parents of a minor and incompetent girl, K.M., petitioned through counsel to be appointed guardians of her person and her estate. They also wanted authorization to consent to her sterilization.

K.M. has an IQ of 40 with a mental age of 6 to 7 years. Her independent functioning is severely limited. K.M.'s neurologist testified that she would never be able to exercise responsible judgment in sexual matters or in caring for a child. K.M. expressed to a counselor that she did not want to have children, but she may have been parroting what she heard her parents say.

The court ruled that K.M. could be sterilized, and her parents were granted authorization. Authorization was withheld pending appeal.

Outcome: Reversed and remanded. The court was found in error for not appointing independent counsel for K.M. Juvenile Law, Case Summaries, re the Guardianship of K.M., No. 25941-5-1 (Division One), September 16, 1991.

Vignette 11

A married couple have five healthy daughters but want a son. The wife is pregnant and wants prenatal diagnosis solely to learn the sex of the fetus. If the diagnosis cannot be made, the wife wants to abort the fetus. Also, if the diagnosis shows the fetus to be female, she wants to abort the fetus. The husband believes that prenatal diagnosis to determine sex is wrong and does not want to consent to the testing. He convinces his wife to abort the fetus without knowing the sex. An abortion was performed, but the wife agonizes and wonders years later if she made the "right" decision.

Note: This vignette was derived from several case studies by Wertz, DC, and Fletcher, JC: Fatal knowledge? Prenatal diagnosis and sex selection. Hastings Cent Rep pp 25–26, May/June, 1989.

Vignette 12

A 33-year-old man works in a local food handling plant in a small northern Minnesota town of 3000. The plant employs approximately 14 people and sells wholesale to the public for the larger surrounding community. The man begins to lose weight, feel weak, and develop coldlike symptoms, which soon cause him to miss days of work. His employer visits him at home to find he is living with another man and has been diagnosed with acquired immunodeficiency syndrome (AIDS). The man is able to work but is weaker.

Before long, the community knows his diagnosis, and the food handling plant loses a significant number of buyers. The employee with AIDS continues to work at the plant when he is physically able. Finally, someone attempts arson on the plant. The arson was an attempt to let the employer know that the community does not want a person with AIDS working in the plant.

Vignette 13

When executing a living will of a 76-year-old man who has been advised to have kidney dialysis, whose authority is paramount when there is disagreement among the nephrologist, the primary care physician, the client, and the family?

Later the same client is on the dialysis machine, and wants to discontinue the machine against the advice of the nephrologist. Has the authority changed?

Would the authority change in either of the two preceding situations if dialysis is performed while the client is a hospital inpatient as opposed to a client in a dialysis center?

Vignette 14

A patient is referred to a consultant for diagnosis. The consultant's receptionist secretary obtains the patient information, including the referring physician's name. The receptionist secretary is not familiar with this doctor's name, looks it up in the telephone directory, and cannot locate any information on the doctor. She comments to the patient, "I cannot find your doctor's name in the directory. He must not be licensed to practice."

When the patient is examined by the consultant, the consultant makes some derogatory comments about the referring physician.

The patient later tells his primary physician what the receptionist secretary and consultant said. *Kaplan v Goodfried*, 497 SW2n 101 (1973).

Vignette 15

When the client, Bass, suffered nausea and complications from the side effects of a tuberculosis drug, he sued the doctor and his assistant because the assistant, Sharon Stone, a CMA, did not inform the client of the side effects.

Outcome: The court ruled that the physician, Dr. Barksdale, not the assistant, was liable because it is the physician's duty to inform the client of complications.

Note: This vignette is based, in part, on *Bass v Barksdale,* 671 SW2d 476 (Tenn App 1984).

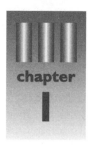

chapter 1

Medical Law, Ethics, and Bioethics

LEARNING OBJECTIVES

Upon successful completion of this chapter, you will be able to:

1. Define the term *law*.
2. Define the term *ethics*.
3. Define the term *bioethics*.
4. Compare the terms *law, ethics,* and *bioethics*.
5. Explain the importance of ethics, law, and bioethics in the practice of medicine.
6. List and discuss at least five ethical codes.
7. Discuss some bioethical issues in medicine.
8. Describe the characteristics that are important in a professional ambulatory health care employee.

DEFINITION

Pluralistic. Referring to numerous distinct ethnic, religious, and cultural groups that coexist in society.

The title *Medical Law, Ethics, and Bioethics for Ambulatory Care* implies three distinct topics: law, ethics, and bioethics. Such distinction, however, is for the sake of clarity. These topics are integrated throughout the text. Discussing health laws without considering ethics and bioethics is nearly impossible. Conversely, discussing ethics and bioethics without considering the law is futile.

LAW

Laws are societal rules or regulations that are advisable or obligatory to observe. Laws protect the welfare and safety of society, resolve conflicts in an orderly and nonviolent manner, and constantly evolve in accordance with an increasingly **pluralistic** society. Laws have governed humankind and the practice of medicine for thousands of years. Today federal and state governments have constitutional authority to create and enforce laws. A brief look at these laws, their sources, and their definitions appears in subsequent chapters.

ETHICS

Ethics is a set of moral standards and a code for behavior that govern an individual's actions with other individuals and within society. Fletcher[1] differentiates *morals* from ethics, stating, "'morality' is what people do in fact believe to be right and good, while 'ethics' is critical reflection about morality and the rational analysis of it." According to Fletcher, for example, "Should I terminate pregnancy?" is a moral question, while "How should I go about deciding?" is an ethical concern.[1]

Although laws are more apt to be universal rules observed by all, different cultures have different moral codes. Therefore there are no universal truths in ethics because it is difficult to say that customs are either correct or incorrect. Every standard for ethics is culture bound. A person's personal code has no special status; it is only one among many.

Ethics also refers to the various codes of conduct that have been established through the years by members of the medical profession. These codes appear in the appendixes.

BIOETHICS

Bioethics refers to the moral issues and problems that have arisen as a result of modern medicine and research. *Bio* refers to life, and issues in bioethics are often life-and-death issues. Ethical and bioethical standards can be personal, organizational, institutional, or worldwide.

The change in ethics related to modern medicine and research in the past decades is most intriguing. Medicine and technology rapidly change and offer choices to clients and their families. The public is more informed and knowledgeable in the field of bioethics. The public has come to a time of "moral critique" wherein bioethics are not only something read about, but lived on a daily basis.[2] Bioethics provide challenges, excitement, and choices, albeit difficult, for each of us.

During President Clinton's first term, he established an 18-member National Bioethics Advisor Commission (NBAC) with the charge to provide advice and to make recommendations to the National Science and Technology Council (NSTC) and other appropriate agencies on bioethical issues related to research. The NBAC came about once disclosures related to Cold War radiation experiments were known. The appointment ended 13 years of silence imposed by the previous two presidents. The NBAC is an avenue for debate on topics such as informed consent, genetic tissue storage, and human embryo research.

ETHICAL ISSUES IN MODERN MEDICINE

Many situations arise in the practice of medicine and in medical research that present problems requiring moral decisions. A few of these can be illustrated by the following questions.

Should a parent have a right to refuse immunizations for his or her child? Is basic health care a right or a privilege? Does public safety supersede an individual's right? Who dictates client care—the client, the physician, the attorney, or the medical insurance carrier? Should children with serious birth defects be kept alive? Should a woman be allowed an abortion for any reason? Should everyone receive equal treatment in medical care? Should people suffering from a genetic disease be allowed to have children? Should individuals be allowed to die without measures being taken to prolong life? Should criteria be developed to determine who receives donor organs?

None of these questions has an easy answer, and one hopes never to have to deal with them. However, one may sometimes have to make these decisions or be in a position to assist those who make such decisions. These questions and possibilities are the reason for including a discussion of pertinent bioethical issues.

We do not attempt in this book to determine right or wrong for the ethical issues in modern medicine. The purpose is to present the law and the facts that are pertinent in the ambulatory health care setting and to raise some questions for consideration. Most of us have decided what *ought* to be in each of the bioethical issues. That is important. It also is important to know how and why our opinions have been formed and to look at what *is*—in other words, what is acceptable according to the legal and ethical standards of today.

As health professionals we must live and act so that we have respect for ourselves and for others and encourage others to have respect for themselves. We need to know what we are to become and how we can become better than we are. We hope that the forthcoming discussions on "Allocation of Scarce Medical Resources," "Genetic Engineering," "Abortion," "Acquired Immunodeficiency Syndrome," "Life and Death," and "Dying and Death" will offer a better understanding of what *is* and what may *become*. The chapter "Have a Care!" and the Epilogue will better define for you who we are as authors and what we have become in writing this book.

In reading the following chapters and considering their effect on you personally as well as your role as a health professional, you may find the following lines from a poem by F.A. Rollo Russel (1849–1914) helpful.

> Seek the right, perform the true,
> Raise the work and life anew.
> Hearts around you sink with care;
> You can help their load to bear.
> You can bring inspiring light,
> Arm their faltering will to fight.

COMPARING LAW, ETHICS, AND BIOETHICS

Law, ethics, and bioethics are different yet related concepts. Laws are mandatory rules to which all citizens must adhere or risk civil or criminal liability. Ethics often relate to morals and set forth universal goals that we try to meet. However, there is no temporal penalty for failing to meet the goals as there is apt to be in law. Laws are seen by many as being "too blunt, as scaring people unnecessarily, as interfering, and as counterproductive."[2] Yet most could agree that law in the United States has been the driving force in shaping our ethics.

Confusion over the definitions of law, ethics, and bioethics is understandable. Consider the following example for further clarification.

The U.S. Supreme Court addressed the issue of abortion. In law it ruled that during the first trimester, pregnant women have a constitutional right to abortions, and the state has no vested interest in regulating them at this time. During the second trimester, the state may regulate abortions and insist on reasonable standards of medical practice if an abortion is to be performed.[3] During the third trimester, the state interests override pregnant women's rights to abortions, and the state may "proscribe abortion except when necessary to preserve the health or life of the mother."[4]

The personal ethics of a physician or health care professional may dictate nonparticipation in an abortion or any abortion-related activities.

Bioethics and the allocation of scarce resources are evidenced by some state statutes that have denied the use of state funds for an abortion. As in this example, sometimes law, ethics, and bioethics conflict.

▄▄▄ THE IMPORTANCE OF MEDICAL LAW, ETHICS, AND BIOETHICS

"Why are medical law, ethics, and bioethics necessary?" is a reasonable question. To offer an adequate answer, one must consider the climate of medical care today. Factors relevant to this climate include the following:

1. Demands of society for quality health care at a minimal personal cost
2. The debate over whether health care is a right or a privilege
3. The equality of the distribution and access to emerging medical technology
4. The controversy among managed care, the political arena, and the consumer about who pays and how
5. The potential for greed among all participants in health care
6. The powerful role of medical insurance and managed care

Almost daily, consumers are bombarded with information on medicine and health care. The media, both printed and electronic, report on some aspect of health care. This immediate access to information causes consumers to ask more questions of the medical community and to expect to be well informed about choices. Ethical standards and laws designed to protect clients and establish guidelines for the medical profession are efforts to create a climate for an equitable exchange between client and provider. Increasingly, ambulatory care centers are establishing ethics committees that enable community resource persons, educators, and providers to grapple with ethical dilemmas before they occur in the clinical setting. The goal of such an ethics committee is to have a plan in place before a crisis occurs.

Medical technology is advancing at a more rapid rate than either laypersons can comprehend or legal or ethical standards can address. Consider the developments in reproductive techniques. Years ago, when a woman wanted a baby, her options were readily defined. Now, with continual advancements in medical technology, her options have greatly increased. A woman desiring a child also can be impregnated artificially. Such choices have their advantages and disadvantages. What influence should the doctor have in presenting these choices to the mother-to-be? Are there any problems for an offspring? Who should be involved in the decisions? Do state laws differ regarding such matters? Ambulatory health care employees need to be aware of the ethical and legal implications of such choices.

Medical specialization means more people will be involved in personal health care. Managed care, policies, and providers will in part dictate how choices are made. If hospitalization is necessary, two or more specialists may be called. Who coordinates and approves this care? Who decides the appropriate course of action in the case of conflicting medical opinions? Although specialization may enhance quality health care, it demands greater coordination for clients to benefit from it, and it increases the cost of medical care.

In 1940 a normal delivery cost a couple $35 for 10 days of inpatient hospital care. The delivering physician received an additional $35. In 1990 a normal delivery cost an average of $3300 for a 2- to 3-day inpatient hospital stay. Poll your fellow classmates and friends for today's costs of a normal delivery, and a radical philosophy change will also be noted. In 1996 Congress forced health insurance to provide a minimum of a 48-hour hospital stay for normal delivery.

By the year 2000 it is estimated that 60 million Americans will be without health services.[5] Medicare and medicaid now pay less of the total bill for the elderly and the indigent than was originally planned, and a large population of working poor who hold down one or more part-time jobs do not qualify for medical benefits. At the same time, managed care is instituting every cost-saving measure possible, thus dictating to providers what and how costs will be covered.

For example, a 47-year-old man requiring surgery for a hernia reported to the hospital operating room in the morning and was discharged to his home the evening of the operation because his insurance would not cover an overnight stay. His wife, untrained in nursing care, had to take 2 days' leave from work to care for him. As the burden of quality health care costs begins to shift back to consumers, we can expect to see more states passing laws regarding the equitable distribution of health care dollars and additional ethical concerns raised over that distribution.

Oregon's Basic Health Care Services Act of 1989 sought to expand coverage and access to health care by extending medicaid eligibility to most Oregonians below the federal poverty line. Further, the law identified basic health benefits for all persons in the state.[6] The problem, of course, is the realization that in providing basic health care for all Oregon residents, choices were made identifying those procedures that are to be covered and those to be eliminated (see Chapter 12).

CODES OF ETHICS

Professional codes have evolved throughout history as practitioners grappled with various ethical and bioethical issues. Increasingly, groups of professionals have defined how members of their profession ought to behave. Complete transcripts of the various codes to be considered can be found in the appendices at the end of the book, but a brief summary of each follows.

The Hippocratic oath, although not prominent in medical schools today, still may be found on the walls of many ambulatory health care settings and clinics. The oath, which was first written in the fifth century BC, became Christianized in the 10th or 11th century AD to eliminate referral to pagan gods. The Hippocratic oath protected the rights of patients and appealed to the inner and finer instincts of the physician without imposing penalties.

The Geneva Convention Code of Medical Ethics, established by the World Medical Association in 1949, is similar to the Hippocratic oath. This code refers to colleagues as brothers and states that religion, race, and other such factors are not a consideration for care of the total person. This code reflects the fact that medicine was becoming available to all during this era.

The Nuremberg Code was established between 1946 and 1949 as a result of the trials of war criminals after World War II. This code suggests guidelines for human experimentation and is directed to the world. The writers hoped that the code would ensure the safety of humans in the years to come.

The Declaration of Helsinki, written between 1964 and 1975, is an update on human experimentation. Much more detailed than the Nuremberg Code, it includes guidelines for both therapeutic and scientific clinical research. Unlike the Nuremberg Code, the Declaration of Helsinki is directed to the world of medicine rather than the world at large.

The Code for Nurses was adopted by the International Council of Nurses in 1973. It is a more general code and refers to an idealistic lifestyle and basic standards of nursing care.

The Medical Assistant Code of Ethics is similar to the code of nursing ethics except that it is directed to the medical assistant and to office and clinic assisting rather than nursing. The code, revised in 1996, was adopted by the American Association of Medical Assistants and appears in its constitution and bylaws.

The American Medical Association established the Principles of Medical Ethics in 1847 and updated it in 1957 and 1980. The Preamble and Seven Principles have served as guidelines for physicians for many years. The document "Current Opinions of the Judicial Council of the American Medical Association" is intended as an adjunct to the revised Principles of Medical Ethics.[7] Both documents are pertinent to physicians and their assistants today.

Other codes have appeared that deal more with the rights of clients than the responsibilities and guidelines for health care providers. They include the Patient's Bill of Rights, presented by the American Hospital Association in 1973. The purpose of this document is to inform clients of rights they have always had but of which they may not have been aware.

█████ AN ETHICS CHECK

Blanchard and Peale,[8] in *The Power of Ethical Management,* developed a set of questions to serve as an "ethics check" that is a useful tool for persons facing an ethical dilemma. The ethics check suggests that ethics is a very personal concept and personal decision.

A personal code to adopt might include Blanchard and Peale's three questions:

1. Is it legal or in accordance with institutional or company policy?
2. Does it promote a win-win situation with as many individuals (client/employee/employer) as possible?
3. How would I feel about myself were I to read about my decision or action in the daily newspaper? How would my family feel? Can I look myself in the mirror?[8]

If the answer to any one of the three questions is no, the action is unethical. If the answer to all three questions is yes, the action is ethical. The clarification of our own personal code of ethics helps clarify actions; however, these ethics check questions might further clarify how we should act when in a difficult situation.

An individual will have great difficulties remaining ethical in an organization that is unethical. It helps if the leader of a group is ethical, making it easier for everyone else to be ethical. However, ethical actions may come from anyone regardless of status.

CRITICAL THINKING EXERCISE

You are the office manager in a large multiphysician medical center. There is no upward mobility in this center, and you relish a new challenge. It is a rather slow day, and you use your office computer to access the Internet to do a job search. You find four that are exciting, and you send your resume on the Internet. As you close out of the Internet, you recall that it is easy to trace access sites on the Internet. Apply the ethics check.

CHARACTERISTICS OF A PROFESSIONAL AMBULATORY HEALTH CARE EMPLOYEE

The significant conflict that often arises among law, ethics, and bioethics mandates that individuals choosing health professions be persons of high moral standards. They should be clear, open, and knowledgeable about their personal choices and beliefs and be able to recognize vast diversity in a pluralistic society. Health care professionals must feel comfortable in a "servant" role while maintaining their own integrity and the respect of their clients.

Individuals employed in a service-oriented industry such as health care are expected to have certain characteristics. The health professional must always be tactful and should know instinctively when speaking is wise and when listening is better. The ambulatory health care employee is an important communication link between the client and the physician.

Clients expect to be treated with courtesy and understanding. Only the most caring and sensitive of employees can handle day after day of sick, hurting, and complaining clients and remain objective yet compassionate.

Physician employers require that their employees be diligent and knowledgeable in every detail of the job. Such knowledge and training can come only through professional preparation that is demanding and exacting and that is continued throughout employment.

Honesty and integrity are traits required of the employee. Physicians' employees must remember to practice only within the scope of their professional training and under the direct supervision of the doctor. Confidentiality must be tenaciously protected, and both the clients' and the physicians' best interests must be guarded. (Refer to Vignette 1, which presents an example

Vignette 1

A certified medical assistant (CMA) employed by an obstetrician/gynecologist calls her former medical assistant instructor to inform her of an opening for a clinical assistant in the obstetrics and gynecology (OB/GYN) clinic. After describing the position and its responsibilities, the CMA says, "We really need another person in the clinical area. I'm the doctor's only nurse."

Surprised by the comment, the instructor inquires, "When did you go back to school to become a nurse?"

She replies, "Oh, I didn't, but everyone thinks I am his nurse. I do everything a nurse does."

of a certified medical assistant who calls herself a "nurse," yet she is not a nurse.)

Wise and prudent ambulatory health care employees will select employers for whom they have respect and to whom they can remain loyal. Matching your personal understanding of "standard of care" to that of your employer avoids conflicts at a later time.

The majority of health care professionals have a concern for quality health care, and that concern is often reflected in community efforts and contributions.

Persons who have these traits are successful ambulatory health care employees who will find their profession rewarding and fulfilling. There is no opportunity for boredom in such a fast-paced and rapidly changing field as health care.

REFERENCES

1. Fletcher, J: The Ethics of Genetic Control Ending Reproductive Roulette. Prometheus Books, Buffalo, NY, 1988, pp xiii–xiv.
2. Annas, GJ: Ethics committees from ethical comfort to ethic cover. Hastings Cent Rep 21:18, 1991.
3. Hemelt, MD, and Mackert, ME: Dynamics of Law in Nursing and Health Care, ed 2. Reston, Boston, 1982, pp 115–116.
4. Mohr, JC: Abortion in America: The Origins and Evolution of National Policy 1800–1900. Oxford University Press, New York, 1978, p 249.
5. Koop, CE: Manage with care. Time 148(14):67, 1996.
6. Doughtery, CJ: Setting health care priorities: Oregon's next step. Hastings Cent Rep 21:3, 1991.
7. Code of Medical Ethics: Current Opinions of the Council and Judicial Affairs of the American Medical Association. American Medical Association, 1996, p xiv.
8. Blanchard, K, and Peale, NV: The Power of Ethical Management. Wm Morrow, New York, 1988, p 27.

BIBLIOGRAPHY

Aiken, T, and Catalano, J: Legal, Ethical, and Political Issues in Nursing. FA Davis, Philadelphia, 1994.
American Medical News: Summaries for Aug 26, 1996, Professional Issues.
Faden, R: The Advisory Committee on Human Radiation Experiments: Reflections on a presidential commission. Hastings Cent Rep 26(5):5, 1996.
Ferrell, OC, and Fraedrich, J: Business Ethics. Houghton Mifflin, Boston, 1997.
Phillips, DF: Ethics consultation quality: Is evaluation feasible? JAMA June 26, 1996.
Rodwin, M: Medicare Money and Morals. Oxford University Press, New York, 1993.
Washington Weekly. The Rutherford Institute, Jan 16, 1997. National Bioethics Advisory Commission meets in Washington, D.C.

Discussion Questions

1. State in your own words what ethics, law, and bioethics mean to you, and give an example of each.

2. What is the difference between law and ethics? Can a law be unethical? Can an ethic be unlawful?

3. What would you do if your ethics do not agree with those of your physician employers?

4. Why is an understanding of bioethics important?

5. Do the Medical Assistant Code of Ethics and the Principles of Medical Ethics have any conflicting views?

6. In a small group discussion, determine the three most important characteristics for a professional ambulatory health care employee. Defend your choices.

Medical Practice Management

LEARNING OBJECTIVES

Upon successful completion of this chapter, you will be able to:

1. Define the types of medical practice management.
2. List two advantages and two disadvantages of each of the types of practice management for both the physician and the employee.
3. Compare personnel needs in each of the types of practice management.
4. Describe managed care options.
5. Define the term *health maintenance organization (HMO)*.
6. Discuss HMO options.
7. Discuss joint ventures and preferred provider organizations.
8. Define the concept of general liability for physicians.
9. Identify physicians' responsibilities to employees in medical practice management.

DEFINITIONS

Bond. An insurance contract by which a bonding agency guarantees payment of a specified sum to an employer in the event of a financial loss caused the employer by the act of a specified employee; a legal obligation to pay specific sums.

Burglary. Breaking and entering with intent to commit a felony.

Capitation. Health care providers are paid a fixed monthly fee for a range of services for each HMO member in their care.

Conglomerates. A corporation of a number of different companies operating in a number of different fields.

Co-payment. A medical expense that is a member's responsibility; usually a fixed amount of $5 to $20.

Deductible. A cost-sharing arrangement in which the member pays a set amount toward covered services before the insurer pays. Typically, HMO members do not pay deductibles.

Fee-for-service. Pay providers receive for each service performed.

Gatekeeper. A term referring to HMO primary care physicians or nurse practitioners responsible for referring members to specialists with the intent of matching the client's needs and preferences with the appropriate and cost-effective use of those services.

Group practice. Type of business management in which three or more individuals organize to render professional service sharing the same equipment and personnel.

Health maintenance organization (HMO). Prepaid health care services rendered by participating physicians to an enrolled group of persons.

Liability. Legally bound or obligated, as to make good any loss or damage that occurs; responsible.

Opt-out option. Members or clients can seek treatment from providers outside the health care plan but pay more to do so.

Partnership. Type of business management involving the association of two or more individuals who are co-owners of their business.

Preferred provider organization (PPO). A type of business agreement between a medical service provider and an insurer organization in which the fees for specific services are predetermined for an already established group of patients assigned and/or selected to the provider.

Professional service corporation. Specific type of corporation in which licensed individuals organize to render a professional service to the public. Such licensed individuals include physicians, lawyers, and dentists.

Sole proprietorship. Type of business management owned by a single individual.

Theft. Actual taking and carrying of someone else's personal property without consent or authority and with the intent to permanently deprive a person of it.

Physicians have traditionally practiced as sole proprietorships, as partners with other physicians, as members of health maintenance organizations (HMOs), and as shareholder/employees in professional service corporations. Increasingly, however, many physicians practice in a complicated combination of more than one type of medical practice management. Which type of business management to select is an early decision made by physicians entering practice but may change throughout one's career.

Even though the business organization may change from time to time and dictate a change in certain legal questions, the physician employer, like any other employer, incurs general **liability** for the activities of the business. General liability includes making good any loss or damage related to the business such as liability for **theft** or fire and the safety of employees and premises.

A change in medical practice management will have an impact on the ambulatory health care employees and their work. The change will be seen in medical records, billing and accounting procedures, payroll, number and duties of employees, and benefits. Office employees need to be aware of how the type of business organization affects them and their jobs.

▬ SOLE PROPRIETORS

A **sole proprietorship,** or single proprietorship, is a business owned by a single individual who receives all the profits and takes all the risks (Fig. 2–1). It is the oldest form of business and is the easiest to start, operate, and dissolve. Even sole proprietors, however, are likely to function in one or more health maintenance insurance programs as preferred providers. Physicians serving as sole or single proprietors of their ambulatory health care settings will find advantages and disadvantages to this form of business management.

Advantages of Sole Proprietorships

The advantages of a sole proprietorship include simplicity of organization; being one's own boss; being the sole receiver of all profits; and having fewer government regulations, low organizational costs, and great flexibility in operation.

To illustrate the advantages of the sole proprietorship, consider the example of a doctor who is able to establish a practice in a community by purchasing or renting facilities, to make decisions without consideration of partners or other business colleagues, and to incur minimal organizational costs. The doctor also will not have to divide the profits with any

Sole Proprietor

FIGURE 2–1. Graphical representation of a sole proprietor.

other person and will be able to run the practice exactly as desired. When participating as a preferred provider in an HMO, however, the physician must follow the guidelines of the HMO but does have free choice on whether to participate.

Disadvantages of Sole Proprietorships

There are disadvantages, however, to the single proprietorship. For instance, physicians may have difficulties raising sufficient capital to begin or expand the business. Medical equipment is among the most expensive of any type of equipment in a new business. The profits of the business may be insufficient to allow for expansion. Also, physicians must know that if the business fails in a single proprietorship, their personal property may be attached, and they may lose virtually all personal savings and possessions. The sole proprietor typically performs all or most of the managerial functions in the business and works more than a standard 40-hour workweek.

Consider again a doctor who has sufficient capital when entering practice to establish the office as a sole proprietorship. Initially, the system works well while the client load is light. However, the doctor soon finds that time is at a premium when working 70 to 80 hours a week carrying a full client load and managing the business aspects of the practice as well.

Considerations for the Ambulatory Health Care Employee

The sole proprietor will probably begin with just one assistant. This person will need training in all areas of administrative and clinical tasks to be performed in the ambulatory health care setting. Although some assistants enjoy the opportunity to use all their skills in the whole operation, others may find this situation less attractive and prefer that the physician allow certain tasks to be sent outside the office for completion. These tasks might include laboratory work, transcription, correspondence, or billing and coding. The sole proprietorship often uses the services of an accountant for quarterly and yearly tax reports.

The sole proprietorship offers little if any opportunity for advancement for its employees. Therefore the physician has to reward employees with pay raises and benefits to encourage them to remain as employees or bear the expense of hiring and retraining a new employee. Physicians will select employees carefully on the basis of their education, training, and experience; reward them sufficiently for their work; and encourage them to stay a long time with the practice. Many office assistants may prefer the sole proprietorship because of the opportunity they have to make decisions and assume leadership responsibilities.

PARTNERSHIPS

A **partnership** is an association of two or more persons who are co-owners of a business for profit (Fig. 2–2). Most partnerships have only two or three members, but there is no limit to the number of individuals who may enter into a partnership. The organization may take many forms and should be defined in a partnership agreement.

The agreement should be written and reviewed by an attorney. It should include such items as the kind of business to be conducted or services to be performed, the kind of partnership being established, authority held by each partner, length of the partnership agreement, capital invested by each partner, description of how profits and losses are to be shared, how each partner is to be compensated, limitations on monetary withdrawals by a partner, accounting procedures to be followed, procedures for admitting new partners, dissolution of the partnership, and, of course, the signatures of the partners involved in the agreement.

Advantages of Partnerships

Some advantages of partnerships are easily recognized. Generally, a partnership has more financial strength than a sole proprietorship. Partners are likely to bring additional managerial skill and a sharing of the workload. The organization of a partnership remains relatively simple, although somewhat more complicated than a sole proprietorship.

When a doctor is deciding how to establish a practice, the partnership may be desirable. If the practice is already established, only a small capital investment may be required in the beginning. This investment can be increased as the doctor becomes more financially secure. A sole proprietor often will turn to a partnership when the workload of the practice requires a second person to share the work.

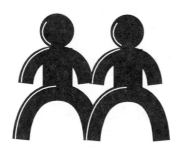

Partnership

FIGURE 2–2. Graphical representation of a partnership.

Disadvantages of Partnerships

A disadvantage of a partnership is that two or more people make the decisions. A partner cannot be the only "boss." In addition, each partner is responsible for the business. If one partner lacks the personal finances to assume a full share of any loss, the other partners are required to make good the deficit. If the partnership fails, usually one partner can be liable for the whole amount of the partnership debts, regardless of the size of the investment.

Personality differences should be considered because compatibility is important in any partnership. A trial period that allows a partner to withdraw from the association or be asked to withdraw after a given period may be advantageous.

If the doctor does not wish to enter a partnership agreement but needs additional help, another physician may be hired strictly on a salary basis. Although this arrangement does not constitute a partnership, a contract may be desirable for the protection of each party.

Considerations for the Ambulatory Health Care Employee

A partnership should consider hiring more than one assistant in the ambulatory health care setting because of the increased workload. Each partner may desire an assistant, but many tasks will be common to each and are best performed by one person. Assistants must understand the partnership relationship and the line of authority. Open communication on the part of all members of the staff is essential. Otherwise, each physician may expect an assistant to function as a member of the staff but may not provide input as to how this should be done.

In addition, with more than one employee, both job advancement and job specialization are possible. For example, the newly formed partnership hiring a second assistant may want to name the first assistant office manager with a specific set of duties or to assign one assistant to administrative tasks while the other performs clinical duties.

▬ PROFESSIONAL SERVICE CORPORATIONS

A corporation is a legal entity that is granted many of the same rights enjoyed by individuals (Fig. 2–3). These include the right to own, mortgage, and dispose of property, the right to manage its own affairs, and the right to sue and be sued. Physicians in a **professional service corporation** remain personally liable for their acts of medical malpractice.

Professional service associations or professional corporations are designed for professional persons such as physicians, lawyers, dentists, and ac-

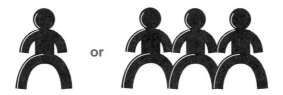

Professional Service Corporations

FIGURE 2–3. Graphical representation of a professional service corporation.

countants. These corporations can be identified by the letters SC (service corporation), PC (professional corporation), PSC (professional service corporation), Inc., (incorporated), and PA (professional association), depending on state law. The professional service corporation is the most intricate of all forms of medical practice and can be formed for one or more individuals.

Advantages of Professional Service Corporations

Advantages of professional service corporations include the fact that contributions to pension or profit-sharing plans can be made for all employees, including the physician. Such funds are deducted by the corporation from its taxable income, are invested, and accumulate in tax-free trusts until a future time of disbursement. Taxes are not paid on the funds until the time of their disbursement, usually at retirement, when the individual is in a lower tax bracket.

Another advantage is the corporate medical reimbursement plan. Medical and dental expenses are deductible to the corporation and nontaxable to the employee. This can result in substantial savings to both corporation and employee. Group term life insurance on a deductible premium basis is another advantage of a professional corporation. The professional corporation also may pay the professional liability premiums for physicians and their employees. Furthermore, in a corporation, physicians' personal assets are protected and cannot be attached to satisfy a debt as they can be in a sole proprietorship or partnership.

Disadvantages of Professional Service Corporations

When professional service corporations first became legal, many physicians eagerly incorporated, only to discover the disadvantages. The complexity of the professional service corporation and its detailed requirements call for reliable, well-informed attorneys and accountants to advise the corporation. The professional service corporation may be more expensive to operate than other forms of organization.

Physicians in professional service corporations have discovered that full participation in pensions, profit-sharing plans, and medical reimbursement plans is essential if the full benefits of this form of organization are to be realized. Regular meetings and agreement on organization, investments, pensions, and profit-sharing plans are important and legally required. Because more individuals are involved than in a sole proprietorship or most partnerships, decision making is more complicated. Physicians often have problems finding the time to perform the functions required to run a corporation.

Although a professional service corporation usually involves two or more physicians functioning in a group setting, a sole proprietor can incorporate as a professional service corporation. The income of a single individual who incorporates needs to be sufficient to allow full participation in the benefits granted to the professional service corporation or such an arrangement is financially ineffectual.

Considerations for the Ambulatory Health Care Employee

The professional service corporation generally employs more assistants than a partnership or sole proprietorship. The possibility of being a part of a profit-sharing plan and having medical expenses covered by the corporation is an attractive inducement to prospective employees. This form of practice usually provides ample opportunity for advancement and specialization. One person should be responsible for all personnel matters to enable a smooth-running organization.

▪▪▪ GROUP PRACTICES

Another option of medical practice available to physicians is joining a **group practice** (Fig. 2–4). The physician in group practice will either be a partner, an officer of the corporation, or an employee of the practice. Most group practices are corporations, but as the workload increases, new physicians often are hired as employees. The American Medical Association (AMA) defines group practice as follows:

> Group medical practice is the application of medical services by three or more physicians formally organized to provide medical care, consultation, diagnosis, and/or treatment through the joint use of equipment and personnel, and with the income from medical practice distributed in accordance with methods previously determined by members of the group.[1]

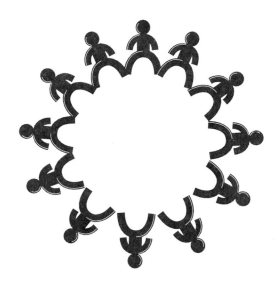

Group Practice

FIGURE 2–4. Graphical representation of a group practice.

There are three main types of group practice:

1. Single specialty, providing services in only one field of practice or major specialty; for example, a group of pediatricians joining together in practice
2. Multispecialty, providing services in two or more fields of practice or major specialties; for example, a group of obstetricians/gynecologists and pediatricians joining together in practice
3. Primary care group, providing services by obstetricians/gynecologists, pediatricians, family practitioners, and internists

Group medical practices operate on a **fee-for-service** basis, through insurance coverage, HMO or preferred provider arrangements, or even private pay with the same type of business arrangement as a sole proprietorship, a partnership, or a professional service corporation.

Advantages of Group Practices

Advantages to physicians in group practice include a shared financial investment for diagnostic and therapeutic equipment, the opportunity for consultation with other physicians, little administrative responsibility for the practice (a group may actually employ a medical manager for the business side of the operation), and more family and recreation time because physicians in the group cover for one another. In addition, group practice may offer the intellectual and social stimulation desired by some physicians.

Disadvantages of Group Practices

The disadvantages of group practices are easily identified. Not every physician has the personality to function well in a group setting. A physician cannot act totally independent of the group and may feel a loss of freedom in such a situation. Although the working hours may not be as long as in solo practice, the income also may not be as high. Working in a close relationship with colleagues on a daily basis may lead to personality clashes and differences of opinion.

Considerations for the Ambulatory Health Care Employee

A group practice will have more employees than the other forms of medical organization simply because of the larger staff of physicians. Physicians generally will have less responsibility for hiring and selecting personnel, which may be an advantage or a disadvantage, depending on the physician's personal preferences. An employee may choose employment in a group for many of the same reasons as those in the corporation. Depending on the number of employees, a larger group may be less personalized.

MANAGED CARE

In recent years, a form of management called managed care has experienced rapid growth (Fig. 2–5). Although it is not a form of management, managed care has dramatically restructured the delivery and financial aspects of health care. No physician can practice without feeling the effects of this system. Clients, too, may question whether they are being treated as a "customer" or as a person. Some question the managed care corporations about their financial interest in managed care. Practical information is needed to address ethical concerns that arise in the context of managed care. To fully understand managed care, a brief history of insurance coverage is warranted.

In the early 1900s consumers expected to pay for all health care from their own pockets. During the depression, many health care providers received little or no pay for their services. Blue Cross first provided insurance for hospital costs in the early 1930s. Blue Shield was introduced soon afterward to cover office and physician costs. Both were driven by union activity in the automobile industry.

Soon employees expected that a part of their employment benefit package would include health insurance to cover all but a few incidental and

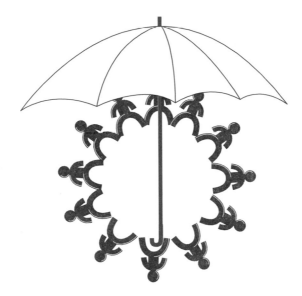

Managed Care

FIGURE 2–5. Graphical representation of managed care. Note that the umbrella covers and protects the individuals involved.

minor expenses. Increased specialization, advancing technology, and little or no emphasis on preventive care drove health care costs to a new all-time high. Employers began to struggle with the increased costs of offering health insurance to an all-demanding workforce. Health maintenance organizations (see p. 33) were introduced to emphasize preventive health care, assure physicians they would receive payment for their services, and ultimately begin to contain costs. It was not long before nearly every insurance carrier was offering some form of an HMO.

Not all physicians and health care consumers were excited about HMOs, however. In some cases, consumers lost the right to choose any primary care physicians. The choice had to be made from a list of participating physicians. A complaint of physicians was the loss of control in the physician-client relationship. While the Health Security Bill to provide basic health care to all persons was being hotly debated in Congress and across the country, HMOs continued to grow in popularity by paying close attention to preventive care, standardizing many medical practices, and eliminating unnecessary tests and procedures. The Health Security Bill was rejected by Congress in 1994, but managed care marched on.

The method of payment for professional services changed. Instead of the fee-for-service method of payment, in which a provider is paid for each service rendered, the **co-payment, deductible,** and **capitation** methods became popular.

The deductible requires policyholders to pay a set amount toward covered services on a fee-for-service basis before the insurer pays claims. Physicians, however, often receive only a percentage (80–90%) of the cost of their services once the insurer's responsibility begins.

Co-payments, a specific dollar amount paid by the client or member (usually $5–$20), were established. The co-payment helped clients realize their responsibility toward payment but is not an amount considered too exorbitant. The co-payment adds a cash flow to the provider receiving deductible amounts and the percentage paid by insurers for remaining services.

Another method of payment, much less popular with providers, and little known and understood by clients, is capitation. Capitation gives health care providers a fixed monthly fee for a range of services for each HMO member under their care rather than a fee for each service performed. The average capitation fee per client in 1997 was between $25 and $35 per month.

One can readily see the complexity of the problem faced by both providers and consumers in understanding the payment process and the cost of health care.

What were seemingly subtle changes in the managed care contracts has had a great impact on physicians and clients. Many found themselves in a form of managed care in which profit rather than health was the motive. Increasingly, physicians must contact a third party for permission to perform certain procedures or make a referral to a specialist. Likewise, a client's health care services are completely paid for if obtained from a preferred provider chosen by the insurance carrier but only partially paid if obtained from an unaffiliated provider. This is known as a **preferred provider organization** (PPO). Further, some managed care plans allow members to seek treatment outside the network but charge the members more to do so. This is called an **opt-out option.**

The problems of a business-first, client care–second system are not only in managed care insurances. Covered fee-for-service plans have similar problems. The increased power of insurance carriers, who no longer just collect premiums from subscribers and process claims, continues to take decision making away from physicians and clients. In 1997 President Clinton appointed a 32-member health care commission to explore growing concerns from consumers that the quality of medical care is declining as costs of medical care are cut. The commission's role is to write a consumer's "bill of rights" to protect the growing number of persons enrolled in HMOs and other managed care plans, as well as the traditional fee-for-service arrangements. President Clinton's charge to the commission (whose report is scheduled to be submitted by March, 1998) is that doctors must be able to discuss all medical options with their clients and to ensure that caregivers are not rewarded for not giving care.

▨▨▨ HEALTH MAINTENANCE ORGANIZATIONS

The **health maintenance organization** is a dominating form of medical practice management in today's society (Fig. 2–6). Kaiser Foundation Health Plan, with over 6 million members, is the largest HMO in the country. It is estimated that about 47 million people belong to an HMO nationwide. In this form of management, groups contract with clients to provide comprehensive health care and preventive medicine for prepaid fees that entitle the subscriber to service during the duration of the contract.

The staff-model HMO owns and operates health care centers staffed by providers employed directly by the plan. These health care centers provide a broad range of services under one roof.

Another form of HMO allows physicians to maintain their private practices, charge their fee-for-service clients, and be reimbursed for the prepayment clients by a central HMO organization. The physicians involved in this form of HMO may have clients who have prepaid for their services to any number of HMO organizations that will, in turn, pay the physician. The HMO may make use of the concept of primary care physician (often referred to as a **gatekeeper**) as a method of controlling costs where all medical care sought by a client must be channeled through the primary care physician.

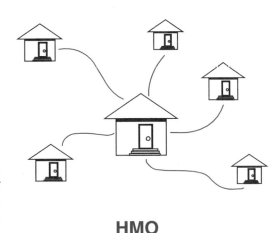

FIGURE 2–6. Graphical representation of one form of health maintenance organization (HMO). Note how the satellites extend from the main provider.

HMO

The advantage to physicians who practice in a staff-model HMO is that the working hours will be regular and allow the physician more personal time. Also, such a physician will not have to provide the building or equipment necessary for practice.

Generally speaking, published research on health care quality shows that HMO members are more satisfied with their care than are members with other forms of coverage. Compared with fee-for-service health insurance, HMO clients received more preventive care, received treatment earlier, and achieved medical outcomes equivalent to or better than fee-for-service medicine. For example, from the Internet Home Page of the Massachusetts Association of HMOs, a recent poll of Massachusetts residents revealed that 79% of HMO members would recommend their health care plan to friends or relatives, compared with 50% of members of fee-for-service plans.

Some form of managed care or managed competition seems destined to play a role in the health care delivery system for some time to come. Good and bad HMOs and managed care plans are no different from good and bad health care providers. Change will most likely come from informed clients who will benefit most from their health care providers. Information available through television, public service programs, and print and electronic media will empower clients by giving them the information and vocabulary necessary to make themselves true partners in the physician-client relationship.

OTHER BUSINESS ARRANGEMENTS

Today's ambulatory health care setting as a form of business management for medical practice is rapidly changing. In cities and their surrounding areas, fewer physicians are sole proprietors. However, the physician as sole proprietor may still be found in the more rural areas of the country. Larger clinics, professional service corporations, and **conglomerates** are increasingly popular.

Joint Ventures

Competition, marketing, and escalating costs have encouraged hospitals and physicians to enter into joint ventures that may be profitable and advantageous to both entities. For example, hospitals are building ambulatory health care settings within their service area to entice physicians to rent the offices and in turn refer their clients to the hospital (Fig. 2–7). Hospitals may purchase a practice and staff it with one or more of their physicians. Such ventures provide physicians with improved marketing capabilities and fewer start-up costs.

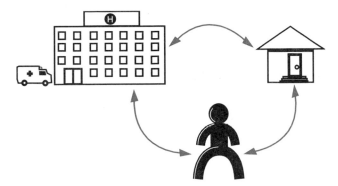

FIGURE 2–7. Graphical representation of a joint venture. Note how all parties are interrelated.

Physician-hospital organizations (PHOs) combine hospital and group medical practices in order to offer clients a "one-stop shopping approach." A primary reason in forming a PHO is the concept that combined services are more attractive than either would be alone. Additionally, both physicians and hospitals benefit one another. Clients receive more services, sometimes at a lower cost. This concept is becoming increasingly popular.

The multiple service organization (MSO) can be owned by physicians, hospitals, a totally separate party, or any combination of the three (Fig. 2–8). This organization is developed to perform physician office management services. For example, the MSO often provides secretarial and office services, billing and collections, group purchasing, and computer servicing. An MSO allows physicians to focus on client care and permits the management service to run the business side of the organization.

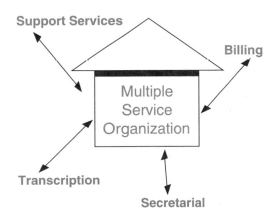

FIGURE 2–8. Graphical representation of a multiple service organization.

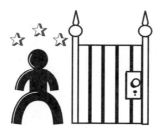

Preferred Provider

FIGURE 2–9. Graphical representation of a preferred provider.

Preferred Provider Organizations

A physician may be a sole proprietor, a partner, or a member of a professional service corporation, as well as a preferred provider for an organization (Fig. 2–9). This arrangement is a contractual agreement between an insurer organization and the physician to provide medical care to an already established number of clients. For example, a physician may contract with Blue Cross's preferred provider plan to give medical care to a certain number of individuals who have subscribed to the Blue Cross preferred provider plan.

▬▬ A WORD OF CAUTION

Physicians considering a move into any of the integrated organizations should be certain that the business arrangement does not violate antitrust laws. Antitrust laws exist to preserve free market competition. Consequently, under antitrust laws any activities that restrict competition are seen as unfavorable.

Physicians must ensure that the business arrangement does not oppose medicare's fee-for-service reimbursement rules or violate any medicare or medicaid fraud and abuse laws. For example, because medicare seeks a direct relationship with its providers, it may not recognize some business organizations as being eligible for medicare reimbursement. Medicare and medicaid laws further prohibit kickbacks and some referrals. For example, physicians cannot refer medicare or medicaid clients to any entity in which they have any financial interest.

More and more physicians are entering into a variety of business management arrangements; however, physicians must seek the appropriate legal advice to ensure that they are within the legal bounds of medical practice.

CRITICAL THINKING EXERCISES

The sole proprietor, age 60, is distraught by the direction medicine is taking. His 70-year-old, otherwise healthy client is scheduled for a double hernia operation but will have less than a 24-hour hospital stay. The physician laments, "This is not the kind of medicine I want to practice."

In a joint venture arrangement, the hospital manages three satellite clinics. In one of the clinics, there is concern that a physician assistant (PA) is spending too much time with clients. The PA is asked to log time in and time out for clients seen over a 3-week period. The PA's profitability is in question.

The large medical conglomerate provides services to health care providers in rural areas that would otherwise not have access to medical specialists. For example, a physician in a rural area can send her electrocardiograph over the phone lines and have it read by a cardiac specialist, resulting in state-of-the-art, immediate diagnosis and treatment.

GENERAL LIABILITY

Physicians engaged in business must be aware of their general liability, which includes liability for building, automobile, theft, fire, and employees' safety.

Office employees will be involved in payments of insurance premiums and submission of claims or in the establishment of physicians in practice. An understanding of the physician's general liability will be a helpful asset to any employee.

Business License

Some communities require a business or occupational license before allowing an office to be opened for the practice of medicine. Physicians should check with county and city clerks to determine whether a license is required and what procedures are to be followed. An annual renewal fee may be necessary.

Building

The physician or the organization that owns the building is responsible for the building and grounds where business is conducted. If a person is injured on those premises, physicians may be held legally responsible. Therefore physicians and managing organizations carry liability insurance for the premises.

Automobile

Aside from personal car insurance, physicians may want to consider nonowner liability insurance. Such a plan protects the physician employer if an employee has an automobile accident while performing some duty related to the business. For physicians who commonly ask their employees to make a bank deposit on their drive home or to deliver the monthly statements to the post office, such protection is wise. Whose car an employee drives makes no difference.[2]

Theft, Fire, and Burglary

Physicians should have protection against theft, fire, and **burglary** on the building, as well as on equipment and furniture. Two types of fire insurance are most common. A co-insurance plan dictates that the owner is responsible for payment of a certain percentage of the loss, such as 20 or 30 percent. A second plan covers not only the loss but also the replacement costs. The latter is, of course, more expensive, but more beneficial in the case of loss.

Cost of protection from burglary and theft depends on location and the amount of money or valuables kept on the premises. Large amounts of money should not be kept in the office, even though most burglary attempts are made for the purpose of taking narcotics. A discussion with insurance agents will identify proper protection.

Some physicians may also insure their accounts receivable, which would be nearly impossible to recover in case of fire or loss. These items belong in a fireproof cabinet or safe after working hours to prevent their loss, even if insured.

Employee Safety

Physicians are expected to provide a safe place of employment for their employees. Safety requirements vary from state to state. Some of the variables include the number of employees, the type of employment, and the safety record of the business. Check with the state agency administering such safety regulations and workers' compensation statutes and with the state medical association to determine responsibility in this area. Refer to Chapter 10 for a discussion of regulations to protect employee safety.

Bonding

Physicians may wish to **bond** employees who are handling financial records and money in the ambulatory health care setting. Bonding is an insurance contract with a bonding agency. The purchase of a bond for a certain amount in an employee's name ensures that physicians will recover the amount of the loss, up to the amount of the bond, in case the employee embezzles funds. This precaution may be especially important when physicians do not have the time to spot-check financial transactions made by employees. Careful employers ask prospective employees if they are bondable.

▬ EMPLOYERS' RESPONSIBILITIES TO EMPLOYEES

Whatever the style of operation in which physicians choose to practice, there are certain business responsibilities for employers. These include federal, state, and local requirements for Social Security compensation protection and workers' compensation for all employees. Benefits can include uniform allowance, paid parking, medical benefits, retirement benefits, profit-sharing plans, vacations, sick leave, paid holidays and personal leave time, professional improvement allowances, and professional liability insurance.

As stated previously in this chapter, physicians must realize the value of appropriately qualified and educated employees and encourage employees to remain with the organization as long as possible. Specific information about physicians' responsibilities to employees can be obtained from an accountant or attorney. County or state medical associations have information about requirements for setting up a practice and also have guidelines for employees. The AMA booklet *Enhancing the Value of Your Medical Practice* and the AMA publication *Group Practice Kit* can be ordered from AMA, Order Department, PO Box 109050, Chicago, IL 60610-9050.

▬ SUMMARY

Physicians can open new practices, function as sole proprietors, be employed by other physicians on a straight salary basis, establish partnerships, become part of professional service corporations, and practice alone or in groups. Most also will be related to some form of HMO and participate in more than one form of managed health care. All forms of medical practice have advantages and disadvantages. The choice depends on the individual personality and preference of the physician. None should be entered into without advice and consideration from persons knowledgeable in the field. The overriding factor for physicians to consider is what type of business organization will best permit them to serve their clients. Physicians must remember that the type of practice chosen will dictate their responsibilities in all areas of general liability. To be less than meticulous in this area of business potentially mars a physician's reputation.

REFERENCES

1. American Medical Association: The Business Side of Medical Practice. AMA, Milwaukee, Wis, 1989, p 6.
2. Ibid, p 48.

BIBLIOGRAPHY

DeVaro, E, and Turner, L: Research Notes: Values in Managed Care. Hastings Cent Rep 27(1):48, 1997.
Furrow, BR, et al: Health Law, Vol. I. West, St Paul, Minn, 1995.
Health Security: The President's Report to the American People. Washington, DC, The White House Domestic Policy Council, 1993.
Koop, CE: Manage with care. Time Fall, 1996.
The HMO Locator: Overview of HMOs in America. MedAccess Corporation, 1996. (Available on Internet for all parts of the country: http//www.medaccess.com/hmos/hmo 01.htm.)
Thomas, D: Positioning Your Practice for the Managed Care Market. Williams & Wilkins, Baltimore, 1996.

Discussion Questions

1. *What kind of business management exists in the ambulatory health care setting where you are employed or where you would be most interested in seeking employment?*

2. *Give reasons why physicians may choose a particular style of business management at different stages of their careers.*

3. *You are offered a position in an HMO but enjoy your present position in a sole proprietorship. What must you consider in making a decision?*

4. *You are convinced that medical costs must be contained but are not certain that the HMO is the answer. What are the alternatives?*

5. *What would the functions of the bookkeeper entail in an ambulatory health care setting in which the physician was a preferred provider for many separate insurers?*

6. *Why would a physician in an ambulatory health care setting or clinic have the bookkeeper bonded?*

7. *List areas of concern that the issue of managed care raises.*

chapter 3

The Employees in Ambulatory Health Care

LEARNING OBJECTIVES

Upon successful completion of this chapter, you will be able to:

1. List and define the four categories of ambulatory health care employees.
2. List and define the three categories of nurses found in an ambulatory health care setting and compare their education and training.
3. Provide at least three examples of nonlicensed personnel in an ambulatory health care setting.
4. List two similarities and dissimilarities between (1) a technician and a technologist and (2) a physician assistant and a medical assistant.

DEFINITIONS

Certification. Documentation, usually from a professional organization, that an individual has met certain requirements set forth by that organization.

Endorsement. An agreement in which one state recognizes the licensing procedure of another state, considers it valid, and grants a license to a physician to practice. Sometimes referred to as reciprocity.

Licensed practical nurse (LPN); licensed vocational nurse (LVN). Person who has graduated from a 1-year practical nurse vocational or college program and has passed the state licensing examination for practical or vocational nurses. An LPN or LVN works under the direct supervision of a registered nurse (RN) or a physician.

Licensure. Legal permission, granted by state statutes, to perform specific acts; as a physician is licensed to practice medicine.

Medical assistant (MA). Person who assists the physician in both administrative (front office) and clinical (back office) duties; education varies from on-the-job training to 2 years in an accredited program for medical assisting. May be certified (CMA) or registered (RMA) by successfully passing the professional organization examination.

Medical laboratory technician (MLT). Person who has graduated from a certificate program or associate degree program and then works under the supervision of a physician or medical technologist in a laboratory. May be certified by a professional organization examination.

Medical technologist (MT). Person who has graduated from a 2- to 4-year college or university program in medical technology that includes 1 year of clinical training in the laboratory.

Nurse practitioner (NP). An RN who has successfully completed additional training in an NP program. An NP can function alone or under the supervision of a physician in a medical facility.

Physician assistant (PA). Person with 1 to 4 years of education in an approved program for PAs; a PA works under the license and supervision of a physician.

Reciprocity. An agreement by which two states recognize the licensing procedures of each other, consider them valid, and grant licenses to practice based on the other state's licensure. In some states, it is referred to as endorsement.

Registered nurse (RN). Person who has graduated from a 2-year associate degree, 3-year diploma, or a 4- to 5-year bachelor's degree program and passed the state licensing examination for RNs. An RN works under the direction of a physician.

Registration. An entry in an official record listing names of persons satisfying certain requirements.

The number and kinds of employees in the ambulatory health care setting vary with the practice. Generally, the more specialized the practice, the more specialized the personnel. Employees in the ambulatory health care setting may fall into the following categories: (1) those who are licensed, (2) those who are registered, and (3) those who are certified. Some employees may be none of the three, and some more than one.

Licensure is the strongest form of regulation. Licensed employees must obtain their licenses from the state authority before employment. A license establishes that the employee has met minimum standards required by law. Licensure of physicians is discussed in Chapter 5.

Registration is a process by which individuals in a particular health field are listed in a registry. This list is then available to health care providers. The state has little or no power over the registration process. There are two method of registration. One occurs when individuals list their names in an official register of a health area in which they work. There is no power to deny employment to unlisted persons, however. The second requires a certain level of education or payment of a fee for registration.

Certification probably is the most common form of regulation. It occurs when a particular organization warrants that the certified person has attained a certain level of knowledge and skill, generally through examination. Again, however, this does not prevent anyone without certification from practicing.

Licensed, certified, and registered persons may use appropriate symbols after their names to verify their credentials. Examples include the RN (registered nurse), CMA (certified medical assistant), and MT (ASCP) for medical technologist (American Society of Clinical Pathologists). Both certification and registration are voluntary. Licensure is mandatory.

People who are not licensed, registered, or certified are also employed in ambulatory health care settings. There is no professional organization regulating these employees. They may be trained on the job, or they may have professional training and education but have not attained certification or registration.

▇▇ LICENSED PERSONNEL (NURSES)

Training and education for nurses fall into three categories: **licensed practical nurse (LPN)** or **licensed vocational nurse (LVN)**, **registered nurse (RN)**, and **nurse practitioner (NP)**.

Licensed Practical Nurse; Licensed Vocational Nurse

Graduate practical nurses (GPNs) may take a state board examination to be licensed as an LPN or LVN. The GPN has completed a 1-year vocational education course at a community agency; a public vocational school; or a junior, community, or senior college. The substance of this program includes elementary nursing practices and introductory educational courses. This nurse is considered a technician.

Registered Nurse

Graduate nurses (GNs) from one of three types of educational programs must take the state board examination to be licensed as an RN.

1. The diploma nurse is generally a graduate of an accredited hospital-based program of 2 or 3 years during which nurses engage in client care and classroom work. Direct client care and bedside experience are stressed.
2. The associate degree nurse is a graduate of an accredited junior or community college program that awards graduates an associate degree in nursing. The college provides the educational base and condenses the practical instruction into a 2-year program.

3. The bachelor's degree nurse is a graduate of a 4- or 5-year program that stresses the importance of general nursing education rather than hospital-based experience. Most administrative positions are held by bachelor's degree nurses, as are the positions of public health and school nurse.

The GN sits for the same state board examination regardless of educational preparation. The GPN also sits for a state board examination; however, the examination differs from that for GNs. The education and training received in all these programs emphasize hospital or nursing facility employment rather than office employment.

The nurse must pass the appropriate state examination in order to use the LPN, LVN, or RN title. This license is renewed as mandated by state law. Most states require a renewal fee; some states require continuing education units (CEUs) for license renewal. Continuing education includes seminars, workshops, college courses, independent studies, and approved on-the-job training. Nurses must keep a record of all successfully completed continuing education classes and submit proof of completion to the appropriate agency when renewing their licenses. All nurses should know their state's requirements and recommendations. Employers of office nurses should have a procedure for checking licenses annually.

Nurses wishing to practice in another state must seek **reciprocity** or **endorsement** in that state. Reciprocity occurs when one state recognizes the licensing procedure of another, considers it valid, and grants a license to practice based on the other's licensure. If there is no reciprocity process, the nurse must satisfy the state's licensure requirement.

Nurse Practitioner

The NP is an RN (usually with a bachelor's degree) who has successfully completed additional training in an NP program. Education and training for NPs usually last 4 months to 1 year and may lead to a specific diploma or a master's degree. The GNP then seeks national certification, which requires written or oral examination. The American Nurses' Association grants the NP certification.

Nurse practitioners usually function independently in expanded nursing roles according to each state's nurse practice act. They may specialize and be certified in such specialities as pediatrics, geriatrics, midwifery, or emergency room medicine. Nurse practitioners may examine, diagnose, and treat clients, acts formerly performed solely by physicians. This diagnosis and treatment often puts the NP in the center of controversy with physicians.

The employment field for NPs varies. For instance, they may be found in isolated areas of the country managing a clinic and providing total client care, or they may be found in public health in charge of family planning clinics. An NP also may be found in a pediatrician's office responsible for the initial history, examination, and screening of clients who are then seen by the physician.

Physicians may choose to employ nurses in offices or clinics because of their technical expertise in clinical areas. Few nurses, however, have skills relating to the business aspect of the ambulatory health care setting or have the desire to function in that capacity.

▰▱ NONLICENSED PERSONNEL

Generally, most ambulatory health care employees are nonlicensed. These individuals include the **physician assistant (PA)**, **medical assistant (MA)**, medical transcriptionist, **medical technologist (MT)**, and **medical laboratory technician (MLT)**. Education and training vary widely among nonlicensed personnel. Many are certified or registered. All function under the supervision of the physician.

Physician Assistant

Physician assistants are usually totally under the control of the medical licensure board, and they practice with the supervision of the licensed doctors of medicine or doctors of osteopathy who employ them. The PA exercises autonomy in medical decision making and provides diagnosis and therapeutic services. The educational requirements for the PA vary widely, from 1 to 4 years. Some programs require 2 years of undergraduate study in biology and behavioral science with some prior work experience in the health field. Two-year programs for PAs provide clinical and practical components covering anatomy and physiology, pathophysiology, microbiology, pharmacology, and applied behavioral science courses. Four-year programs provide the student with liberal arts and behavioral science courses. Both classroom and supervised clinical instruction are common to 2- and 4-year programs. Among tasks performed by PAs are interviewing clients, taking histories, doing routine physical examinations and laboratory tasks, treating burns, suturing and caring for cuts and wounds, changing dressings, making rounds in the hospital, and prescribing and administering medications, always under the supervision and control of the physician employer. Graduates of accredited programs for PAs may apply to the National Commission on Certification for PAs for examination.

Forty-nine states, the District of Columbia, and Guam have enacted legislation affecting PAs. The laws either reconfirm the physician's authority over the PAs or vest authority in a state agency to establish rules for recognition of PAs.

Physicians may be restricted as to the number of PAs they may supervise to ensure that adequate supervision is available. Physician assistants may be found in many areas. Most work with physicians in private or partnership practices in primary care, but some also work in a variety of hospital settings and in group practices.

Medical Assistant

Medical Assistants are often confused with PAs. Both work under the supervision of physicians, but their duties are distinct. The MA's versatility provides for efficient management of the entire health care setting. Although the MA is a generalist, the role may be highly specific, depending on the duties assigned.

Don Balasa, JD, executive director of the American Association of Medical Assistants (AAMA), defines an MA as "an allied health worker, trained to work in outpatient (ambulatory) setting, under a physician's supervision, who is competent in administrative responsibilities, clinical procedures or both." Further, he states that MAs are "not licensed or seeking licensure, seeking independent practice or a physician assistant."[1]

Educational and training programs for the MA are usually 1 or 2 years in a vocational, community, or junior college awarding a certificate, diploma, or associate degree. Programs include academic courses and clinical experience. Typically, the MA receives training and education in both front office (administrative) and back office (clinical) practice.

Medical assistants may achieve credentialing through two sources. The AAMA offers certification; the American Medical Technologists Association offers registration. Both require successful completion of a national examination that covers all aspects of medical assisting. The certified MA may then use the initials "CMA" after his or her name, and the registered MA may use the initials "RMA" after his or her name.

The Commission on Accreditation of Allied Health Programs (CAAHEP) awards or denies accreditation to medical assistant programs (in addition to many other allied health programs). The AAMA, working in conjunction with the AMA, defines the essential components and standards of quality that educational institutions must follow in educating medical assistants. The CAAHEP is recognized by the U.S. Department of Education.

More and more postsecondary schools are seeking CAAHEP accreditation because effective June 1998, only graduates of CAAHEP-accredited medical assistant programs are eligible to sit for the national certification examination. The AAMA believes this will safeguard the quality of care to the consumer, will ensure the CMA's role in a rapidly evolving health care delivery system, and will continue to promote the identity and stature of the profession.

The training and education of MAs specifically prepare them for employment in the ambulatory health care setting. However, the fact that medical assistants function as multiskilled health care practitioners places them in a strategic position to be called multiskilled health practitioners (MSHP).

> The National Multiskilled Health Practitioner Clearinghouse (NMHPC) defines the multiskilled health practitioner as follows:
>
> > *Persons cross trained to provide more than one function, often in more than one discipline. These combined functions can be found in a broad spectrum of health-related jobs, ranging in complexity from the nonprofessional level, including both clinical and management functions. The additional functions (skills) added to the original health care worker's job may be of a higher, lower, or parallel level.*[2]

The economic and political climate in the health care arena provides opportunities for such multiskilled individuals as medical assistants to meet the increasing demands in any number of areas of the health care delivery system.

CRITICAL THINKING EXERCISE

A medical assistant (MA) and registered nurse (RN) work side by side in a large medical setting. There has been recent downsizing, requiring a shifting of assignments. The RN is angered by the MA appointment to an expansion of duties. There is a significant pay difference between the two salaries. Discuss.

OTHER EMPLOYEES

Other employees in the ambulatory health care setting may include the medical receptionist, medical secretary, medical transcriptionist, bookkeeper, insurance biller, and perhaps laboratory technicians. The tasks performed by these individuals are no less important than the others mentioned. Their training and education vary from on-the-job training to formal university education. Three disciplines are specifically identified here. They are the certified medical transcriptionist (CMT), MT, and laboratory technician.

The CMT is a transcriptionist who has passed the national certifying examination given by the American Association of Medical Transcriptionists. A CMT may be employed in the ambulatory health care setting, but a large clinic is more likely to hire a full-time transcriptionist. A smaller facility may employ a transcriptionist part-time or on a contract basis as the need arises. Increasingly, medical transcriptionists are employed in multiservice organizations.

This rapidly growing profession is increasingly in demand. Some community and junior colleges and vocational schools are offering the necessary education and training. Many receive on-the-job training, especially if they have a solid background in medical terminology, possess excellent writing and grammar skills, and are accurate typists.

Medical technologists and MLTs are nonlicensed personnel who may be found in the ambulatory health care setting. The difference is that MTs require little to no supervision and often supervise technicians. Medical technologists can perform complex analyses, fine-line discrimination, and error correction.

Educational requirements for the MT include 4 years of academic studies in a college or university and clinical training. The curriculum includes instruction in hematology, serology, clinical chemistry, microbiology, computer technology, immunohematology, and immunology, emphasizing basic principles commonly used in diagnostic laboratory tests.

Medical laboratory technicians may also be found in ambulatory health care. Education is obtained through either a certificate program or an associate degree program varying in length from 12 to 24 months.

■■■ CONSIDERATIONS FOR AMBULATORY HEALTH CARE EMPLOYEES

All employees of ambulatory health care need to continue their education, regardless of their initial educational preparation. Obviously, continuing education benefits not just the individual and the employer but also, and more important, the welfare of the clients they serve.

State regulations vary and will continue to change as medicine becomes more specialized. In some states, MAs cannot perform venipuncture. Some states also regulate who can practice radiography and who can administer medications. All states regulate laboratory procedures and protocol. A physician employer must understand regulations pertinent to those individuals in his or her employ. Employees also have the professional responsibility to understand regulations pertaining to their jobs. Practicing within the law is essential for the protection of all concerned.

Employers must recognize that hiring employees with appropriate qualifications and credentials will help ensure that clients receive the optimal level of quality care. At the same time, this also helps keep the cost of health care at a suitable level.

SUMMARY

When considering the education and training of various allied health professionals, one must remember that each is a vital link in the chain to quality health care. No one functions independently of any other. Each health professional has skills and responsibilities to complement every other health professional. When competition and territoriality cause conflict between professionals, quality health care is diminished. The education, training, and scope of practice for each allied health professional are specifically and purposefully designed to complement rather than to conflict.

REFERENCES

1. Balasa, DA: Medical assisting: An important ally of medicine in the current legislative environment. PMA 23:22, 1990.
2. Balasa, DA: Growing demand for MSHPs expands opportunities for the medical assisting profession. PMA 28:15, 1995.

BIBLIOGRAPHY

American Medical Association: Allied Health and Rehabilitation Professions Education Directory, 1996–1997. AMA, Chicago, 1996, p 40.

Discussion Questions

1. Case A: *A solo family practitioner is setting up a practice in a small, rural community.* Case B: *Six physicians are entering a group practice in a city of 40,000. Specialties include obstetrics/ gynecology, family practice, internal medicine, and pediatrics. What number and kinds of employees would you recommend in case A? In case B? Explain your choices.*

2. *What kind of medical practice is most likely to use (a) a PA and (b) an MA?*

3. *Discuss the differences between licensure, certification, and registration.*

4. *Research the AAMA definition of an MA. Expand that definition to include tasks that may be appropriately performed in your state.*

Legal Guidelines for Ambulatory Care

LEARNING OBJECTIVES

Upon successful completion of this chapter, you will be able to:

1. Explain in a brief paragraph why knowledge of the law is necessary for ambulatory health care employees.
2. Describe the source of law.
3. List the three branches of government in the United States.
4. Define the following terms: (a) *constitutional law,* (b) *common law,* (c) *statutory law,* (d) *administrative law,* (e) *plaintiff,* (f) *defendant,* (g) *felony,* (h) *misdemeanor.*
5. List two similarities and two dissimilarities between criminal and civil law.
6. Review, in diagram form, the process for (a) a civil case, (b) a misdemeanor case, and (c) a felony case.
7. List the three steps necessary for obtaining a narcotics registration.
8. Describe in outline form the office procedure to follow for administering and dispensing controlled substances.
9. List the five schedules of controlled substances and give an example of each.
10. Diagram the federal court system and state court system.
11. List two factors that determine in which court a case is heard.
12. List two similarities and two dissimilarities between a subpoena and a *subpoena duces tecum.*
13. Explain, in your own words, the trial process.
14. Name two circumstances calling for an expert witness.

DEFINITIONS

Administer a drug. To introduce a drug into the body of a client.
Appellant. One who appeals a court decision to a higher court.

Arraignment. The procedure of calling someone before a court to answer a charge.

Civil case. Court action between private parties, corporations, government bodies, or other organizations. Compensation is usually monetary. Recovery of private rights is sought.

Closing arguments. Summary and last statements made by opposing attorneys at a hearing or trial.

Controlled Substances Act. Federal law regulating the administration, dispensing, and prescription of particular substances that are categorized in five schedules.

Court of appeals. Court that reviews decisions made by a lower court; may reverse, remand, modify, or affirm lower court decision. No live testimony.

Criminal case. Court action brought by the state against individual(s) or groups of people accused of committing a crime; punishment usually imprisonment or a fine; recovery of rights óf society.

Cross-examination. Examination of a witness by an opposing attorney at a hearing or trial.

Defendant. The person or group accused in a court action.

Deposition. A written record of oral testimony made before a public officer for use in a lawsuit.

Direct examination. Examination of a witness by the attorney calling the witness at a hearing or trial.

Dispense a drug. To deliver controlled substances in a bottle, box, or some other container to the client. Under the Controlled Substances Act, the definition also includes the administering of controlled substances.

Examination of witness. Questioning of a witness by attorneys during a court action.

Expert witness (medical). Person trained in medicine who can testify in a court of law as to what the professional standard of care is in the same or similar communities.

Felony. A serious crime such as murder, larceny, assault, or rape. The punishment is usually severe.

Higher or superior court. The court to which appeals of trial court decisions can be made; a court with broader judicial authority than a lower or inferior court.

Judge. A public official who directs court proceedings, instructs the jury on the law governing the case, and pronounces sentence.

Jury. Six to twelve individuals, usually randomly selected, who are administered an oath and serve in court proceedings to reach a fair verdict on the basis of the evidence presented.

Law. Rule or regulation that is advisable or obligatory to observe.

Litigation. A lawsuit; a contest in court.

Lower or inferior court. Usually, the court in which a case is first presented to the trial court; a court with limited judicial authority.

Misdemeanor. Type of crime less serious than a felony.

Opening statements. Statements made by opposing attorneys at the beginning of a court action to outline what they hope to establish in the trial.

Plaintiff. The person or group initiating the action in litigation.

Prescribe a drug. To issue a drug order for a client.

Probate court. State court that handles wills and settles estates.

Sentencing. Imposition of punishment in a criminal proceeding.

Small claims court. Special court intended to simplify and expedite the handling of small claims or debts.

Subpoena. An order to appear in court under penalty for failure to do so.

Subpoena duces tecum. A court order requiring a witness to appear and bring certain records or tangible items to a trial or deposition.

Verdict. Findings or decision of a jury.

The US legal system is complex and multifaceted. It can baffle even the most astute citizen. Physicians and members of their staff may be served subpoenas, calling them to court as defendants. They may also be called to serve as expert witnesses. Basically, there is one federal legal system and 50 different and unique state legal systems, all created by federal and state constitutions. Most legal actions pertinent to ambulatory health care occur within the state and local systems.

■ SOURCES OF LAW

Law encompasses rules derived from several sources. The Constitution of the United States provides the highest judicial authority. Adopted in 1787, it provides the framework for our government. The Constitution, federal law, and treaties take precedence over the constitutional law of the states. The Constitution of the United States is a legal document that defines the structure and function of federal, state, and local government. The federal government has three branches: (1) the legislative branch is the lawmaking body, that is, Congress; (2) the executive branch is the administrator of the law and includes the president; and (3) the judicial branch is the judges and courts, including the Supreme Court. Each branch provides a system of checks and balances for the other two. For example, the power of lawmaking belongs to Congress, but the president can veto its legislation and the judiciary is empowered to review legislation. Congress, in turn, can investigate the president and control the appellate jurisdiction of the federal courts. No one branch has absolute authority. In addition to the federal government, each state has a constitution defining its own specific governing bodies. All powers not conferred specifically on the federal government are retained by the state, yet states vary widely in their assumption of that power.

TYPES OF LAW

There are two basic types of law: common law and statutory law. Common law was developed by judges in England and France over many centuries. It emerged from customs, the ways things were done over time in England and in France. Common law was brought to the United States with the early settlers. Common law, views decided by judges, is always evolving as established principles are tested and adapted in new case situations.

Many of the legal doctrines applied by the courts in the United States are products of the common law developed in England (or in the case of Louisiana, from France). This is a body of law based on judicial decisions that attempts to apply general principles to specific situations that arise. Common law has the force of statutory law, although it is not enacted by the legislature.

Congressional and state legislative bodies enact rules (laws) known as legislative or statutory law. These laws make up the bulk of our laws as they exist today. Publications containing these statutes are known as codes. An example of a statute pertaining to ambulatory health care is a medical practice act, which defines and outlines the practice of medicine in a given state.

Legislative bodies, however, do not have the time or knowledge to enact all laws necessary for the smooth functioning of the government. Thus administrative agencies are given the power to enact regulations that also have the force of law. This type of law is called administrative law. The Internal Revenue Service and Federal Trade Commission are examples of administrative agencies. Both implement extensive rules in their areas of concern.

Administrative law, an extension of legislative law, affects the ambulatory health care employee. The state health department, the state board of medical examiners, and the state board of nurse examiners are administrative agencies that dictate rules and regulations for ambulatory health care. Further, licensing and accrediting bodies, as well as federal government programs such as medicare and medicaid, directly influence many policies, procedures, and functions of ambulatory health care and fall under the category of administrative law. The Drug Enforcement Agency, an administrative agency of the Department of Justice, enforces the Controlled Substances Act.

Civil and Criminal Law

Law may also be classified as civil, criminal, international, and military. International and military law are not considered here. This book concentrates on civil and criminal law because of their importance in the ambulatory health care setting.

CIVIL LAW

Civil law affects relations between individuals, corporations, government bodies, and other organizations. Restitution for a civil wrong is usually monetary in nature. The bulk of law dealt with in ambulatory health care is civil in nature.

In a **civil case,** the party bringing the action (**plaintiff**) must prove the case by presenting evidence that is more convincing to the **judge** or **jury** than the opposing evidence. The procedure for a civil case is shown in Figure 4–1. The plaintiff's complaint is filed in the proper court, usually by an attorney for the plaintiff. The **defendant** is formally summoned, prepares an answer, and files it in the court. If the defendant fails to answer the summons within the prescribed time, the plaintiff will win the case by default and judgment will be entered against the defendant.

Consider, for example, a "slip, trip, and fall" case. Fran enters her physician's office, slips, and falls as she approaches the reception desk. She suffers a simple fracture of the left femur. When the receptionist comes to her aid, they discover that a snag from the rug caught the heel of Fran's shoe. Fran later takes civil action and sues her physician for medical fees and loss of employment wages for the time she was unable to work as a result of her injuries. As the plaintiff, she must prove that her physician (the defendant) was negligent.

The case may be disposed of without a trial. For example, the complaint may be dismissed because of some technical error, the summons may have been improperly served, or the complaint may not have set forth a claim recognized by law. The parties also may decide to settle out of court.

CRIMINAL LAW

Criminal law pertains to crimes and punishment of persons violating the law. Criminal law affects relations between individuals and government. Criminal wrongs are acts against the welfare and safety of the public or society as a whole. Punishment for criminal acts is usually imprisonment or a fine.

A **criminal case** is brought by the state against individuals or groups of people accused of committing a crime. The prosecuting, district, or state

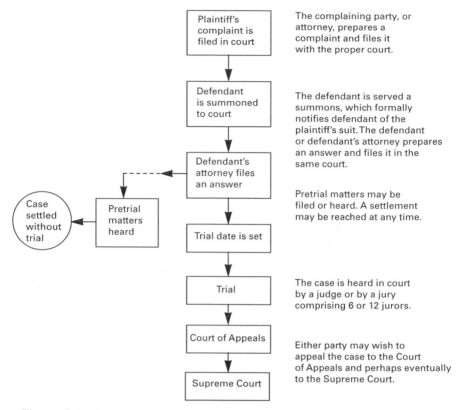

Figure 4–1. Chart explaining the procedure for a civil trial, which helps the public understand the judicial system in that state. Check for similar brochures in your state. (From "A Citizen's Guide to Washington Courts," Washington State Office of Administrator for the Courts, 1993.)

attorney prosecutes the charge against the accused person (defendant) on behalf of the state (plaintiff). The prosecution must prove that the defendant is guilty beyond a reasonable doubt. In other words, the prosecution must be able to prove to the satisfaction of the court that a criminal act was, beyond reasonable doubt, committed by the accused.

A crime is a **felony** or **misdemeanor** that is statutorily defined. Felonies are more serious crimes and include murder, larceny (thefts of large amounts of money), assault, and rape. Gross misdemeanors or misdemeanors are considered lesser offenses. These include disorderly conduct, thefts of small amounts of property, and breaking into an automobile. The misdemeanor and felony case processes are shown in Figures 4–2 and 4–3, respectively.

The procedure for a misdemeanor case is shown in Figure 4–2. The prosecuting attorney is made aware of violations of the law either by traf-

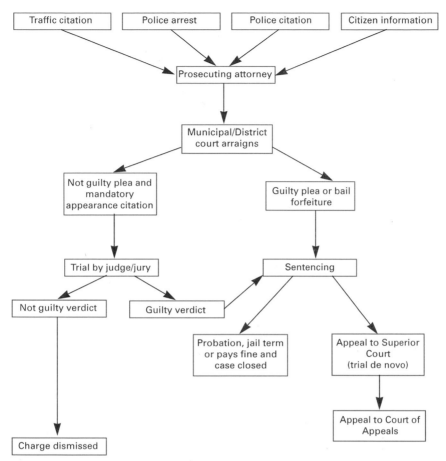

Figure 4–2. Chart of the misdemeanor case process. (From "A Citizen's Guide to Washington Courts," Washington State Office of Administrator for the Courts, 1993.)

fic or police citations, by police arrest, or by citizen information. When the prosecutor determines that enough evidence is present, the court arraigns the person on the prosecutor's charge. The charged person may plead guilty and consequently face **sentencing.** The guilty person may be put on probation, may serve a jail term or pay a fine, or may go through the appellate process. If the charged person pleads not guilty, a trial date is set. At the end of the trial, a **verdict** is given of either guilty or not guilty. If the person is found not guilty, the charge is dismissed. If found guilty, the person faces probation or a jail term or must pay a fine. The guilty person may also use the appellate process (**appellant**).

The felony case process is shown in Figure 4–3. When evidence exists that a crime may have been committed, the police begin their investiga-

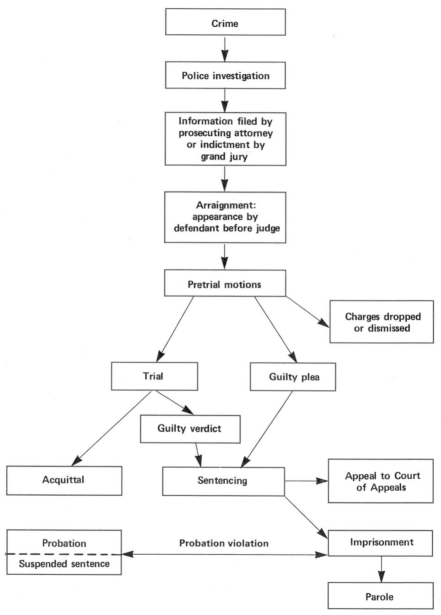

Figure 4–3. Chart of the felony case process. (From "A Citizen's Guide to Washington Courts," Washington State Office of Administrator for the Courts, 1993.)

tion. Then the information is either filed by the prosecuting attorney or given to a grand jury, depending on the practice of the particular jurisdiction and severity of the charge. If the evidence is sufficient, the individual is charged. Pretrial proceedings, to plan the manner in which cases will proceed, are generally informal in nature, and many cases are settled at this point.

If the accused pleads guilty, he or she is sentenced to imprisonment, probation, or a fine. The appellate process then may be available. If the person pleads not guilty, the trial is set, the facts of the case are determined, the principles of law relating to those facts are applied, and a conclusion as to guilt or innocence is reached. If the verdict and judgment are guilty, the individual goes through the same sentencing process as in the guilty plea. If the verdict is not guilty, the person is acquitted.

> ### Where Both Civil and Criminal Law Apply: An Example
>
> To illustrate both civil and criminal law, consider the following situation. Drunk driver Bill is involved in an automobile accident responsible for the death of a homemaker who has two children. Bill is charged by law enforcement officials with involuntary manslaughter and reckless driving while speeding and intoxicated. The courts later find Bill guilty. This is the criminal law protecting society. Taking this situation a step further, the husband of the homemaker sues Bill for a substantial monetary amount to care for the two children, who are now without a mother. On the basis of the facts of the case, the court grants a monetary award. This is civil law.

■■■ CONTROLLED SUBSTANCES ACT AND REGULATIONS

A law all physicians strictly adhere to is the **Controlled Substances Act** regulating addicting medications. Many medications administered, prescribed, or dispensed by physicians do not fall under the Controlled Substances Act. Nevertheless, following federal guidelines for controlled substances when handling other medications is prudent, even though regulations regarding the drugs outside these schedules may be less restrictive.

The Drug Enforcement Administration (DEA) of the Department of Justice is responsible for enforcement of the Comprehensive Drug Abuse Prevention and Control Act of 1970, more commonly known as the Controlled Substances Act.[1] These drugs are controlled because of their potential for abuse and dependence. (Drug abuse is discussed in Chapter 6.) The Controlled Substances Act lists controlled drugs in five schedules (I, II, III, IV, and V), which are discussed in detail later in this section.

The Controlled Substances Act and the *United States Code of Federal Regulations* are important to all physicians but are especially pertinent to those who will **administer a drug, prescribe a drug,** or **dispense a drug** that is listed in the five schedules. Requirement for physicians include registration, record keeping, inventory, and proper security.

Registration is with the DEA, Registration Unit, PO Box 28083, Central Station, Washington, DC 20005. Initial application is made on DEA form 224, which can be obtained from the aforementioned address or any DEA field office. A number is assigned to each legitimate handler, and registration is renewed every 3 years. Generally, a re-registration application is mailed by DEA to the registered physician approximately 60 days before the expiration date of the registration. If the application is not received by the physician within 45 days before the registration expiration, notice of such fact and request for forms must be made in writing to the Registration Unit of the DEA.[2]

A separate DEA registration is granted for each of several business activities and is different for residents, interns, and foreign physicians. Therefore, physicians should check with the DEA to make certain the proper registration is made. The initial registration fee is $20 and must be renewed every 3 years at a cost of $60. The certificate of registration must be readily available at the registration location. Two helpful booklets are the *United States Code of Federal Regulations, Title 21,* parts 1300 to end, revised April 1, 1991, which is available from the Office of the Federal Register, National Archives and Records Service, General Services Administration, and federal government bookstores, and *Physician's Manual,* March 1990, available from the DEA, Office of Public Affairs, and regional DEA offices.

Record keeping and inventorying are required of physicians for the dispensing of narcotic and non-narcotic drugs to clients. The records must be kept for 2 years and are subject to DEA inspection. Inventory must be taken on the date of registration and every 2 years thereafter. The following is required:

1. Name, address, and DEA registration number
2. Date and time of inventory, that is, opening and closing of business
3. Signature of person(s) taking inventory
4. Inventory record to be on file for at least 2 years
5. Separate record required for schedule II drugs[3]

Security is necessary for controlled substances. These drugs must be kept in a locked or double-locked cabinet or a safe that is substantially constructed. Any loss is to be reported to the regional DEA office and local law enforcement.[4]

Physicians who only prescribe narcotic or non-narcotic drugs are not required to keep the detailed record stated previously. State requirements differ, however, and may be more restrictive than federal requirements.

Schedule I

This schedule lists drugs of high potential for abuse and that have no currently accepted medical use. Schedule I drugs can be used by physicians only for purposes of research, which must be approved by the Food and Drug Administration and the DEA, and only after a separate DEA registration as a researcher is obtained.[5] The manufacture, importation, and sale of these drugs is prohibited.

Examples include heroin, marijuana, and lysergic acid diethylamide (LSD).

Schedule II

These drugs have current accepted medical use in the United States, but with severe restrictions. These drugs have a high potential of abuse that may lead to severe psychologic or physical dependence.

Examples of schedule II narcotics include morphine, codeine, and oxycodone with aspirin (Percodan). Examples of non-narcotics include amphetamines, methylphenidate (Ritalin), and sodium pentobarbital (Nembutal).

When these drugs are ordered, the physician must use a special order form that is preprinted with the physician's name and address. The form is issued in triplicate. One copy is kept in the physician's file. The remaining copies are forwarded to the supplier, who, after filling the order, keeps a copy and forwards the third copy to the nearest DEA office.[6]

Prescription orders for schedule II drugs must be written and signed by the physician. Some states, by law, require special prescription blanks with more than one copy. The physician's registration number must appear on the blank. The order may not be telephoned in to the pharmacy except in an emergency, as defined by the DEA. A prescription for schedule II drugs may not be refilled.[7]

Schedule III

These drugs have less potential for abuse than substances in schedules I and II. They have accepted medical use for treatment in the United States, but abuse may lead to moderate or low physical dependence or high psychologic dependence.

Examples of schedule III narcotics include various drug combinations containing codeine and paregoric. Examples of non-narcotics include amphetamine-like compounds and butabarbital.

Schedule IV

These drugs have a lower potential for abuse than those in schedule III and have accepted medical use in the United States, but their abuse still may lead to limited physical or psychological dependence.

Examples include chloral hydrate, meprobamate, chlordiazepoxide (Librium), diazepam (Valium), and propoxyphene (Darvon).

Schedule III and IV drugs require either a written or oral prescription by the prescribing physician. If authorized by the physician or the initial prescription, the client may have the prescription refilled up to the number of refills authorized, which may not exceed five times or beyond 6 months from the date that the prescription was issued.[8]

Schedule V

These drugs have less potential for abuse than drugs in schedule IV, and their abuse may be limited to physical or psychologic dependence. Refills are the same as for drugs in schedules III and IV.

Examples include cough medications containing codeine and antidiarrheals such as diphenoxylate/atropine (Lomotil).

DRUG SCHEDULES

All controlled substances are divided into five schedules. A complete list should be obtained from a regional office of the DEA or can be found in the *United States Code of Federal Regulations, Title 21.* A brief summary is included in the accompanying box.

ISSUING PRESCRIPTIONS

According to the law, the only person authorized to issue prescriptions is the registrant. A prescription issued by the physician may be communicated to the pharmacist by ambulatory health care employees. This regulation may be less restrictive for medications not included in the Controlled Substances Act.

If the state requires triplicate prescription blanks, these will be used for prescribing drugs. These are not to be confused with the DEA form 222 described earlier for the ordering of schedule I and II drugs. The triplicate blanks will be furnished by the state, and the regulations should be followed. For example, in some states, the triplicate blanks may be sequentially numbered.

All prescriptions for controlled substances must be dated and signed on the day issued, bearing the full name and address of the client and the name, address, and DEA registration number of the physician. The prescription must be written in ink or typewritten and must be signed by hand by the physician.[9]

Physicians must also know the laws of their state on controlled substances. The state regulations may be more strict than federal regulations and may require a separate state registration.

Narcotics laws should be studied carefully by any physician who opens an office. The *Code of Federal Regulations, Title 21*, mentioned earlier, should be obtained from the nearest federal government bookstore and studied carefully before controlled substances are handled in the ambulatory health care setting.

■ TYPES OF COURT

As indicated earlier, the type of court that hears a particular case depends on the offense or complaint. In criminal cases, the type of court depends on the nature of the offense and where it occurs. In civil cases, it depends on the amount of money involved and where the parties reside. The jury and judge are neutral arbitrators of the evidence.

Courts also are classified as either lower or higher, inferior or superior. A **lower or inferior court** has less authority than a **higher or superior court.**

Three jurisdictions belong only to federal courts: federal crimes, such as racketeering and bank robbery; constitutional issues; and civil action involving parties not living in the same state. Figure 4–4 illustrates the

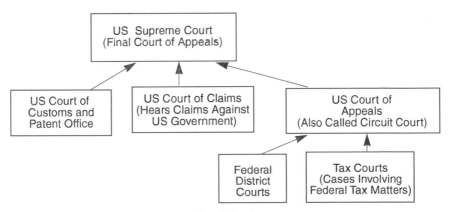

Figure 4–4. The federal court system.

federal court system. The US Supreme Court is the highest court in the federal court system. Directly under jurisdiction of the US Supreme Court are the US Court of Claims, the US Court of Customs and Patent Office, and the US Court of Appeals (or circuit courts). The circuit courts direct the actions of the US Federal District Courts and Tax Courts. In turn, the US Supreme Court directs the actions of all courts: federal, state, trial, and appellate.

The pattern for state courts is similar to the pattern for federal courts. There are inferior or lower courts and a process of appeals.

Figure 4–5 illustrates the state court system. The lower courts hear cases involving civil matters, small claims, housing, traffic, and some misdemeanors. The State Superior Court has general jurisdiction in all types of civil and criminal cases. The **court of appeals** has power to review deci-

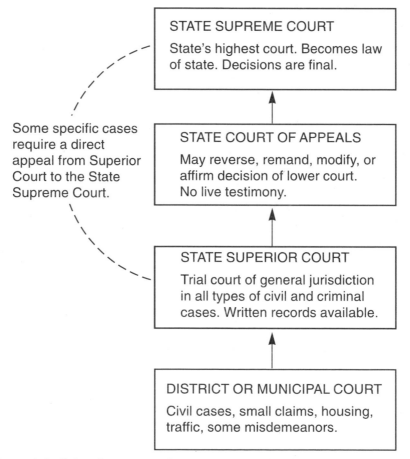

Figure 4–5. Titles of courts vary from state to state, but this diagram illustrates the overall structure of the court system in most states.

sions of this court. The court of appeals may reverse, remand, modify, or affirm a decision of a lower court. The final route of appeal is to the State Supreme Court, the determination of which becomes the law of the state.

Each state defines by statute the types of cases a particular court will hear and the maximum money value of the cases over which it has jurisdiction. In the event litigation does arise, physicians and their ambulatory health care employees most likely find themselves in a state court regarding a civil matter. These civil matters may also take place in **probate court** and **small claims court.**

Probate Court

Probate law oversees the distribution of a person's estate upon death. In probate court (sometimes called estate court), the physician may decide to initiate action on the collection of a bill owed by a deceased client. Generally, the ambulatory health care employee represents the interests of the physician and attempts to locate the responsible person or party for the debt whose name can be obtained from the deceased client's family or lawyer, from the hospital, or from the mortuary. If unable to obtain a name from these sources, the ambulatory health care employee must write or call the county seat in which the estate is being settled. The county probate court recorder will provide information concerning the filing of the claim (in court, to the executor of the estate, or elsewhere), the proper forms to file, and when the claim must be submitted. Quick action is required because most states have a file period of from 4 to 12 months after the publication of notice in a newspaper by the administrator or executor.

Once the probate forms are ready to be mailed, the ambulatory health care employee sends them by certified mail, return receipt requested. This establishes that the documents were received and by whom. The administrator will either accept or reject the claim. If it is accepted, payment will follow, but it may be delayed for months in the courts. If it is rejected and the physician believes the bill is justified, a lawsuit may be filed against the administrator within a designated amount of time, depending on the state. The ambulatory health care employees should be aware of their particular state's time limits.

Keep in mind that even though you may be hesitant to collect a deceased client's bill, the physician rendered services for the client and deserves payment. Failure to file a claim may be construed by others as an admission of poor medical care on the part of the physician.

Small Claims Court

Small claims court allows the physician or physician representative to file action against a client for an unpaid or delinquent account. In addition to the judgment of the amount owed, the physician plaintiff may also recover the costs of the suit. There is no representation by attorney. The plaintiff bringing the action files a preprinted form identifying facts in the account to be collected. A summons is issued on the complaint requesting the appearance of the defendant before the judge.

The defendant is given time to file a cross complaint against the plaintiff for any possible grievance the defendant may have. A date is set for delivery and decision.

The plaintiff presents the facts in the case, and the defendant responds to the allegations or charges. Both parties may **subpoena** witnesses to testify on their behalf. After all information is heard, the matter goes to the judge for a decision. If judgment is in favor of the defendant, there is no right to appeal. However, if judgment is in favor of the plaintiff, the defendant may appeal the decision to a higher court.

The wise ambulatory health care employee will contact the clerk of small claims for instructions and information regarding the procedures to follow in small claims court. This is in direct contrast to lawsuits in higher courts, where court clerks cannot assist the parties in completing forms.

CRITICAL THINKING EXERCISES

How do you protect confidentiality when the office area is in the hallway of a medical facility or when the reception area is very open? How can this lead to a civil case?

Discuss the relationship of anger and litigation; anger on the part of client; anger on the part of the health care professional. For example, if you have a noncompliant client, is anger appropriate?

Although small claims court may be an avenue to collect a client's account, consider the disadvantages of doing so.

SUBPOENAS

Physicians may find themselves in court even though they and their employees have practiced good preventive measures. No matter what the dispute or reason for **litigation,** physicians need to be adequately prepared. The reasons for court appearances are numerous, but most commonly the physician will be a defendant, a witness, or an **expert witness (medical)** in civil or criminal trials; in sanity and probate contests; in personal injury actions; or in cases arising under insurance policies including life, health, or accident.

In any of these cases, physicians may appear with or without a subpoena. A subpoena is a court order commanding attendance in a specific court or office, at a specific time, under penalty for failure to do so unless a protective order from the court invalidates the requirement. See Chapter 8 for an example. The subpoena may be signed by the clerk of the court, a notary public, or an attorney. The subpoena may require a **deposition** to be taken rather than actual appearance in court.

The attendance requested in a subpoena may be of a person (physician or ambulatory health care employee) or of data (medical record). The latter is a *subpoena duces tecum*, which requires the witness to appear and to bring certain records. The physician most likely would not need to appear to identify a record; proper identification can usually be done by an employee. The physician would be necessary, however, to interpret the record.

Whatever the type of subpoena, it should authorize witness fees, photocopying fees, or mileage fees. If fees are not authorized, they are to be requested when the subpoena is served. If the physician is being subpoenaed, the subpoena must be hand-delivered to the physician. However, because so many subpoenas are served and there are so few officers to serve them, some subpoenas may be served to the physician's employee instead of to the physician. In such cases, the physician, out of courtesy, appears in court as though the subpoena was served by an officer to him or her. If the medical record is subpoenaed, the subpoena may be served to an employee. Any questions about a subpoena or its circumstances should be taken to an attorney immediately.

▰▰▰ THE TRIAL PROCESS

A case may be tried before a judge or a judge and jury. Usually, trial courts have a jury, but the parties to a trial may waive (voluntarily give up) their right to a jury trial.

First, the jury, consisting of 6 to 12 people, must be selected. A pool of potential jurors is chosen at random from voter registration lists and auto license records in the area. How the actual jurors are picked from this pool depends on the level of court, the type of case being tried, and local court rules. Once the jurors are selected, they are given the oath by a clerk or judge.

The trial procedure then begins. **Opening statements** usually are made by each attorney, first for the plaintiff and then for the defendant. Such statements outline the facts each party hopes to establish during the trial. The plaintiff's attorney calls the first witness and asks questions (**examination of witness**). This part of the process is called **direct examination**. The defendant's attorney then cross-examines the witness (**cross-examination**). This procedure continues until the plaintiff's entire case has been presented. The case for the defense is presented in the same manner. The direct examinations and cross-examinations recur. In a criminal case, the state must prove guilt "beyond a reasonable doubt," whereas in a civil case it is by a preponderance of evidence. Then both attorneys rest their cases, that is, indicate that no further evidence or testimony is to be given.

If it is a jury trial, the judge then instructs the jury on the law governing the case. The attorney for each party is allowed **closing arguments,** after which the judge charges the jury to reach a fair verdict based on the evidence presented. Then the jury is ushered from the courtroom to consider the case and reach a verdict.

In civil court, the judge or jury finds for the plaintiff or for the defendant. If the verdict is found in favor of the defendant, the case is dismissed. If the plaintiff wins the case, a monetary settlement usually is awarded, the amount determined by the judge or jury.

In a criminal trial, if the defendant is found guilty, the judge imposes sentence. At sentencing, the court can commit the defendant to an institution or allow probation. At the end of the trial, the judge informs the defendant of all rights to appeal. If the defendant is found not guilty, the case is dismissed.

Vignette 2

As a medical assistant educator with several years of experience in the administrative area and a recognized authority on medical records, you have been asked to testify as an expert witness regarding protocol for making corrections in a medical record. You agree.

When you are interviewed by the attorney and given the records to review, you recognize that the person responsible for the data entered in the record is a former student and a practicing certified medical assistant. It appears obvious that the records have been altered after the fact.

◼◼◼ EXPERT WITNESS

In medical cases, an expert witness is a person specifically qualified in medicine who can testify in court as to what the professional standard of care is in the same or a similar community. An expert witness is necessary if the subject of the court action is beyond the general understanding of the average layperson or if the knowledge of the expert witness will aid in discovering the truth.

As expert witnesses, physicians testify as to what they see, hear, know to be fact, and is the recognized standard of care. Opinions not based on their experience or expertise, certain out-of-court statements, and conclusions are not admissible in most cases. Expert witnesses in medical cases are usually skilled in the art, science, or profession of medicine and may be practicing medicine or teaching in a school of medicine. In litigation, attorneys may have difficulty obtaining an expert witness who is geographically close because experts are often hesitant to testify to what may appear to be against their own peers. They are expected to be reputable, honest, and impartial. The attorney who has called the witness will try to establish the witness's training, experience, intelligence, and accuracy. Witnesses should talk in lay terms rather than medical language and bear in mind that their dress and appearance may influence the judge and jury. Attorneys cannot prompt or cue witnesses.

Expert witnesses may wish to illustrate or clarify their testimony by employing visual aids such as videotapes, computer CD-ROM programs, photographs, diagrams, charts, radiographs, skeletons, and human-type models. In some instances, sketch artists or illustrators may be employed. During cross-examination, witnesses may face difficulties. The cross-examining attorney may try to intimidate the witness or create confusion. Witnesses should take their time and answer truthfully. They should not be afraid to say, "I don't know," if that is the case.

Expert witnesses are entitled to a fee commensurate with their time away from their practice or teaching for the case, their preparation for the case, and their participation in the case. If questioned during cross-examination regarding a fee for witnessing, they should answer truthfully. A fee should be established before serving as an expert witness rather than on a contingency basis.

If an ambulatory health care employee or a physician is subpoenaed to be an expert witness, legal counsel should be sought. Ethically such testimony should not be seen as adversarial to peers. An attorney will guide, advise, and take whatever legal action is indicated.

We cannot overstress how important legal counsel is in the case of any questions or doubts. Physicians often seek consultation on difficult medical problems and should do no less for themselves and their employees if faced with litigation.

▰ SUMMARY

This introduction to law does not attempt to provide all the necessary information the ambulatory health care employee may need. It provides basic information, not legal advice. However, ambulatory health care employees must be knowledgeable of the law and aware of their professional responsibilities, especially as they relate to being a defendant or an expert witness. Many activities in ambulatory health care require legal knowledge, and this knowledge of the law may prevent illegal acts.

REFERENCES

1. Drug Enforcement Administration: Physician's Manual. US Department of Justice, Washington, DC, 1990, p 2.
2. Ibid, p 5.
3. Ibid, p 10.
4. Ibid, p 15.
5. Code of Federal Regulations, No. 21, Parts 1300 to end. Office of the Federal Register, Washington, DC, 1991, p 7.
6. Ibid, p 64.
7. Drug Enforcement Administration, p 13.
8. Ibid, p 13.
9. Ibid, p 13.

BIBLIOGRAPHY

Cowdrey, ML, and Drew, M: Basic Law for the Allied Health Professions, ed 2. Jones & Bartlett, Boston, 1995.
Furrow, BR, et al: Health Law. West, St Paul, Minn, 1995.
Medical assistant witness: Self-assessment test. PMA 28(3):11, May–June, 1995.

Discussion Questions

1. *Describe a situation in which an understanding of the law is important to a medical receptionist.*
2. *If you were involved in a civil case, describe the process the case would follow and identify the factors that would determine the appropriate court.*
3. *Is a misdemeanor the same as a felony? Explain.*
4. *A physician from another state is coming into your established practice. What must be done about narcotics registration?*
5. *Currently, are there any cases under consideration in the U.S. Supreme Court that directly affect the ambulatory health care employee?*
6. *When might an expert witness be needed? What suggestions might you have for the witness's court preparation and appearance?*
7. *Clarence calls requesting a refill for oxycodone with aspirin (Percodan). Your records show that he has not been seen by the physician for almost 1 year. The doctor is away from the office for 1 week. What will you do? Consider the legal implications.*

Regulations and Professional Liability for the Health Care Professional

LEARNING OBJECTIVES

Upon successful completion of this chapter, you will be able to:

1. Identify four common requirements for a physician to be licensed.
2. Identify three conditions under which a physician's license may be revoked.
3. Explain professional liability for physicians.
4. Discuss the meaning of standard of care.
5. Discuss confidentiality as related to the standard of care.
6. List three elements necessary for a contract to be valid.
7. Compare and contrast intentional and unintentional torts.
8. Define the terms *negligence* and *malpractice*.
9. Identify the four Ds of negligence for physicians.
10. Define and discuss *res ipsa loquitur* and *respondeat superior*.
11. Define the term *statute of limitations* and identify the three most common points for the statute of limitations to begin.
12. Restate, in your own words, the importance of professional liability insurance.
13. Recall six guidelines of malpractice prevention.

DEFINITIONS

Breach of contract. Failure to comply with the terms of a valid contract.

Defamation. Spoken or written words concerning someone that tend to injure that person's reputation and for which damages can be recovered. Two types of defamation are libel, which is false, defamatory writing, such as published material, effigy, or picture; and slander, which is false, malicious, defamatory spoken words.

"Going bare." Slang term for having no malpractice insurance coverage.

Medical malpractice. Professional negligence of physicians.

Negligence (medical). Doing some act that a reasonable and prudent physician would not do or failing to do some act that a reasonable and prudent physician would do.

Res ipsa loquitur. A Latin phrase meaning "The thing speaks for itself." A doctrine of negligence law.

Respondeat superior. A Latin phrase meaning "Let the master answer"; that is, the physician is responsible for employee acts.

Summons. A court order to appear as a defendant in a case.

Tickler file. A periodic reminder to do specific tasks on schedule; usually daily, weekly, or monthly.

Tort. Wrongful act committed by one person against another person or against property; distinguished from a breach of contract.

Without an understanding of laws that directly relate to physicians, the ambulatory health care employee may inadvertently cause difficulties. Therefore it is important to consider those laws and regulations that directly influence the actions of ambulatory health care employees and physicians.

The law is, at times, both complicated and vague. This book cannot cover all parts of the law as it may affect physicians and employees. Only laws related to the practice of medicine in an office or clinic are emphasized.

One of the greatest fears of employees and physicians in ambulatory health care is the threat of litigation. Caring for persons who may be ill, apprehensive, in pain, or suffering from a terminal condition is risky. Such a risk carries the possibility of litigation, which becomes a reality when a **summons** is served at the ambulatory health care setting on the physician or when someone is subpoenaed to testify in court.

Litigation may be sought for many reasons. A client may sue the physician for **negligence (medical).** Perhaps a contractual arrangement has been violated (**breach of contract**) or a **tort** has been committed.

▨▨▨ MEDICAL PRACTICE ACTS

Medical practice acts are state statutes that define the practice of medicine, describe methods of licensure, and set guidelines for suspension or revocation of a license. All 50 states have such statutes to protect their citizens from harm by unqualified persons practicing medicine.

Licensure

Physicians must be licensed to practice medicine in the United States. States differ in their licensing requirements. The more common requirements include graduation from an accredited medical school, completion of an internship, and successful completion of the United States Medical Licensing Examination (USMLE), which was implemented in 1994. Foreign-trained and foreign-educated physicians are required to pass the USMLE before being allowed to practice in the United States.

Physicians who choose to practice in more than one state must satisfy the license requirements of each state. This may be done by requiring physicians to meet each state's endorsement requirements.[1]

Many states require a complete and unrestricted license to provide medical services. The Department of Defense is encouraging states to require full licensure of its military personnel. Physicians engaging strictly in research and not practicing medicine need not have a license in some states.

License Renewal

Physicians renew their licenses periodically, and payment of a fee is usually required. The physician receives notice at the time of renewal. Documentation of continuing medical education (CME) is commonly a requirement for renewal. Specific state requirements differ. Appropriate credits are identified in the state statutes and may include (1) reading of books, papers, and publications; (2) teaching health professionals; (3) attending approved courses, workshops, and seminars; and (4) self-instruction.[2]

Physicians' employees may be responsible for keeping the records of the continuing medical education activities. To do so, they must have the state's requirements on file and be able to verify the credits as required.

License Revocation and Suspension

A physician's license to practice may be revoked or suspended as a result of (1) conviction of a crime, (2) unprofessional conduct, and (3) personal or professional incapacity. Each of these conditions is defined by state statute.

Conviction of a crime is a more obvious reason for license revocation than is unprofessional conduct or personal or professional incapacity. Examples include physicians who are convicted of child abuse, commit sexual assault against clients, or commit active euthanasia. Unprofessional conduct of all licensed health care professionals, including physicians, generally is defined by law. Although these acts are not crimes, such conduct is unacceptable according to state law and therefore is punishable. Examples of unprofessional conduct include falsifying any records regarding licensing, being dishonest, and impersonating another physician. Personal or professional incapacity includes chronic alcoholism, drug abuse, continuing to practice when severe physical limitations prevent adequate care, and practicing outside the scope of training.

Usually charges against physicians are made by the physicians' licensing board in all three conditions necessitating the suspension or revocation of a physician's license. In all states, the basic procedure for disciplinary action is similar. Most boards are required to give the physician licensee sufficient notice of the charges and allow the physician legal counsel and a hearing. The board then investigates, prosecutes, makes a judgment, and sentences. Some states have empowered their licensing boards to suspend a license to practice on a temporary basis without a hearing when the physician poses an immediate threat. In other words, no due process is necessary if the physician poses an immediate threat.

Vignette 3

A patient seriously injures his thumb and hand on the job. A local physician cleanses and bandages the wound and administers an antitetanus injection. The doctor prescribes antibiotics and pain medication.

The patient is seen by the physician's employee for the next four visits. The medical office employee is a high school graduate who worked approximately 2 years as a nurse's aide in the local hospital before working for this doctor.

On subsequent visits, the employee removes dead tissue and cleanses and bandages the wound. The patient complains of severe pain. The employee expresses pus from the wound on several occasions. The thumb and hand become inflamed, and the patient loses range of motion.

The patient sees the doctor or his employee for 17 more visits during a 2-month period. The employee treats the patient for 12 of the 17 visits.

The patient loses full function of his hand and seeks consultation from another physician. *Delaney v Rosenthall,* 196 NE2d 878 (1966).

PROFESSIONAL LIABILITY

Once physicians become licensed, they become legally liable for their actions as physicians. They are responsible, accountable, obligated, and legally bound by law. Their liability can be either civil or criminal. Criminal liability is less common in ambulatory health care than civil liability. Criminal liability results when an individual commits an act that is considered to be an offense against society as a whole.

Examples of criminal liability for the physician include performing active euthanasia, committing child abuse, and the evasion or breach of the Controlled Substances Act. Physicians found to be grossly negligent or reckless in the death of a client may be held criminally responsible. In some states, the failure of physicians to make certain reports (e.g., child or elder abuse) required by law may be a crime.

Civil liability identifies conflicts between individuals, corporations, government bodies, and other organizations. Examples of civil liability include tort and breach of contract. For example, civil liability occurs when the physician prescribes a pain medication over the phone for a migraine-like headache, not recalling that this person is recovering from hepatitis. Because the pain medication is contraindicated in hepatitis, the person becomes violently ill with resultant liver damage.

STANDARD OF CARE

One cannot fully understand liability without some knowledge of standard of care principles. The acceptable standard of care requires that physicians must use the ordinary and reasonable skill that is commonly used by other reputable practitioners when caring for individuals. They are expected to perform those acts that a reasonable and prudent physician would. The standard also dictates that physicians must not perform any acts that a reasonable and prudent physician would not. Physicians should always practice in the realm of safety and secure all necessary data on which to base a sound judgment. Physicians are expected to exhaust all possible resources available to them when treating individuals. This includes obtaining a thorough medical history, a complete physical examination, and necessary laboratory tests. Physicians are expected to know what new therapeutic developments might benefit those in their care and still not subject them to undue risk.

Employees in ambulatory health care also must adhere to a standard of care. The standard an ambulatory health care employee will be measured against depends on the task the employee is undertaking; the education, training, and experience of the employee; and the responsibility the physician has given the employee. For example, if the ambulatory health care employee is making a diagnosis or treating a client, the employee could be held to the standard of care of the physician. If the employee is acting outside his or her level of competency and the client is injured as a result, the employee could be found negligent. Ambulatory health care employees often act in a variety of roles, and they must understand the standard to which they could be held. If, on the other hand, the ambulatory health care employee is mopping the floor, he or she will be held to the reasonable person standard rather than the standard of a specific health care professional.

CONFIDENTIALITY

Unless otherwise required by law, physicians must keep confidential any communication necessary to treatment of the client. The client's privacy

Vignette 4

Mrs. Farley had a tubal ligation. She was informed of the risks and signed consent forms before surgery. Five months later she returned to the same physician, who determined that she was pregnant. After the birth of Mrs. Farley's baby, the attending physician examined both of her fallopian tubes and found that one was ligated, but the other appeared normal. Mrs. Farley sued the physician who performed the tubal ligation on the basis of res ipsa loquitur.

Outcome: The court held that Mrs. Farley could not rely on the doctrine of res ipsa loquitur to establish the medical malpractice claim against the physician. The court held that "the doctrine of res ipsa loquitur cannot be invoked where the existence of negligence is wholly a matter of conjecture and the circumstances are not proved, but must themselves be presumed, or when it may be inferred that there was no negligence on the part of the defendant." The doctrine only holds in cases in which the defendant's negligence is the only inference that can reasonably and legitimately be drawn from the circumstances. This was not the case here. The court stated that this was probably one of those cases in which the sterilization procedure failed; the ligation was performed, but the ligation band came off soon thereafter. *Farley v Meadows,* 404 SE2d 537 (1991).

must be protected. Physicians and their employees must be extremely careful that all information gained through the care of the client is kept confidential and given only to those health professionals who need to know. Care should also be taken that any information about a client cannot be overheard by others.

Privilege forbids physicians from revealing information about clients in court. Privilege belongs to the client rather than the physician. If a client waives privilege, the physician may not withhold testimony. Not all states recognize the client-physician communication as privileged. The court determines whether the importance of the evidence outweighs any damage caused by disclosure of the information.

■ PHYSICIAN LIABILITY FOR CLIENT INJURY

As early as the 14th century health care professionals have been liable for both contract and negligence principles. A physician-client relationship or contract is normally a prerequisite for litigation against a physician. This is known as contract law. A breach of a contract can bring litigation against a physician. A tort may occur, which is a wrongful act or injury committed by one person against another person (not related to a contract) and for which the court will provide a remedy.

CONTRACTS

Ambulatory health care employees and their physicians are parties to contracts on a daily basis. When a physician accepts a client, a contract has been made. When the office assistant calls an office supply company to reorder office stationery, the assistant acts as the physician's agent in making a contract.

> For a contract to be valid, it must be an agreement between two or more competent people to do or not to do a certain task for payment or for the rendering of a benefit, and the agreement must be lawful.

An example in ambulatory health care occurs when a client calls the office to make an appointment for an annual physical examination. Assuming that the physician is a bona fide physician and the client is a competent adult, the first two parts of the contract exist. The performance of a physical examination is a lawful act, so part three of the contract exists. The client is given a statement of the charges, and the fee is paid. Hence, the contract is valid in all respects.

A contract can be express or implied. An express contract can be written or oral, but all facets of the contract must be specifically stated and understood. An oral contract is as legally binding as a written one; however, it may be more difficult to prove. Physicians' telephone contacts with clients are examples of oral contracts, especially when medical advice is given. A written contract requires that all necessary aspects of the agreement be in writing. Each state, in its statute of frauds, identifies those contracts that must be in writing. Usually included in this list are deeds and mortgages. Most states' statute of frauds includes a section that is pertinent to ambulatory health care, that is, an agreement made by a third party to pay for the medical expenses of another. Such an agreement has to be in writing to be valid. If Elaine tells the medical receptionist that she will pay the medical expenses for her good friend, Diane, the receptionist should ask Elaine to fill out a form to that effect and affix her signature to it.

Implied contracts are the most common form of contracts occurring in ambulatory health care. Such contracts occur every time the physician and client discuss what course of treatment to take and an agreement is reached. An implied agreement does not require a specific expression of the parties involved but is still valid if all points of the contract exist. An implied contract may be implied from the facts or circumstances of the situation or by the law. When a client complains of a sore throat and the physician does a throat culture to diagnose and treat the ailment, a contract is implied by the circumstances of the situation. A contract implied by the law is seen in the example of the physician who administers epinephrine after a client has gone into anaphylactic shock. The law will say that the physician did what the client would have requested had there been an expressed agreement.

Contracts made by the mentally incompetent, the legally insane, those under heavy influence of drugs or alcohol, infants, and some minors are not valid. Such persons are not considered by the law to be competent to enter into binding contracts.

Ambulatory health care employees are generally considered agents of their physician employer. An agent is a person (the ambulatory health care employee) appointed by a principal party (the physician) to perform authorized acts in the name and under the control and direction of the principal. As agents, ambulatory health care employees must be careful of their actions that may become binding on their physician. For example, an employee might promise a cure that in fact is not possible.

The fiduciary obligation on physicians imposed by professional ethics causes courts to look outside the parameters of contract law when determining the physician's obligation to treat a client. Health care professionals are constrained in their ability to withdraw from contractual relationships by judicial case law, which has patient abandonment.

Vignette 5

Kelly, a first-year medical assistant student, tells her instructor that she thinks she may be pregnant and wonders what she should do. The instructor recommends that Kelly go to the campus health center for a pregnancy test. When Kelly's test is positive, she again discusses her case with her instructor. As a single woman, Kelly decides she cannot support a child now but is not sure whether to have the baby and put it up for adoption or to have an abortion. After a few days and a discussion with the father of the child, their decision is to have an abortion.

Kelly returns to the campus health clinic for her test results so that she can take them to the abortion clinic. The certified medical assistant, a former graduate of the school's medical assistant program and a health center employee, refuses to give Kelly the test results, saying "You'll have to talk to the nurse practitioner. I don't believe in abortion." The nurse practitioner gives her the laboratory results.

Abandonment

Once the physician-client relationship has been established, physicians can be found liable if they abandon their clients. To avoid charges of abandonment, the physician should withdraw formally from the case or discharge the client formally. This requires giving reasonable notice to the client with the recommendation for the client to seek further medical care with ample time for the client to secure another physician. This should be done in writing with a copy for the files.

A physician may wish to withdraw from the case if the client fails to follow instructions, take the prescribed medications, or return for recommended appointments. To withdraw formally from a case, a physician should notify the client in writing, state the reasons for the dismissal, and indicate a future date at which the physician is no longer responsible. Such a letter should be sent by certified mail with a return receipt requested. A copy of the letter and the returned receipt are kept in the client's file. To further protect a physician from abandonment charges, all canceled and missed appointments should be noted on the client's chart.

Breach of Contract

A breach of contract arises when one of the parties involved fails to meet the contractual components. For example, the contract may be violated when the client does not pay the bill or refuses to follow medical advice. The contract can be breached when the physician fails to use the treatment promised, promises to use a procedure and then allows someone else to do the procedure, or promises a cure and no cure results. Such breaches of contract are cause for litigation in which the court attempts to make reimbursement to the client for losses suffered. Usually this is in the form of a monetary award.

▌▊▊ TORTS

Tort law is the area of law health care professionals are involved in because it identifies negligence and **medical malpractice.** Medical health care employees or physicians may commit a tort that may result in litigation.

> A tort is a wrongful act committed by one person against another person or against property that causes harm to that person or property. A tort results if there is damage or injury to the client proximately caused by the conduct of the physician or the ambulatory health care employee that does not meet the standard of care governing either the physician or the ambulatory health care employee.

If a physician commits a wrongful act against a client with no resultant client harm, a tort has not been committed.

The two main classifications of torts are intentional and unintentional, or negligence. Intentional torts or wrongs involve the intentional commission of a violation of another person's rights. Unintentional or negligent wrongs are not intentional and may be the result of the omission or the commission of an act. Malpractice is the unintentional tort of professional negligence.

Malpractice is a specific type of negligence that occurs when the standard of care commonly expected from health care professionals is not met. It is also known as professional negligence.

Vignette 6

To continue with the dilemma of Kelly's pregnancy (Vignette 5), consider the following information.

Several days later in the medical assistant clinical class, another medical assistant instructor overhears Nancy, a student who was receiving work experience in the campus health center, breach a confidence and tell other students in the class about Kelly's pregnancy and abortion.

The program's coordinator privately speaks with Nancy about the breach of confidentiality. Nancy responds, "I didn't tell the whole class. I only told my friend."

Professional Negligence or Malpractice

Failure to perform professional duties according to the accepted standard of care is negligence. More specifically, negligence is performing an act that a reasonable and prudent physician would not perform or the failure to perform an act that a reasonable and prudent physician would perform. Negligence, as defined previously, is the same as malpractice. Malpractice may be described as professional negligence.

Professional negligence is more easily prevented than defended. Obviously, physicians do not wish to be found negligent or become involved in a malpractice suit of any kind. However, consumers are more aware of their rights today than ever before. In some cases, clients have been awarded more than 1 million dollars in suits against physicians. Therefore physicians must protect the physician-client relationship at all times and be above reproach in the performance of their duties.

The Four Ds of Negligence

Duty exists when the physician-client relationship has been established. For example, the client calls the office to make an appointment, keeps the appointment, and makes another to return for further treatment.

Derelict is more difficult to define. The client must prove that the physician failed to comply with the standards required and dictated by the profession.

A report of the Committee on Medicolegal Problems of the American Medical Association (AMA) states:

> *To obtain a judgment against a physician for negligence, the patient must present evidence of what have been referred to as the "four Ds." The patient must show: (1) that the physician owed a duty to the patient, (2) that the physician was derelict and breached that duty by failing to act as the ordinary, competent physician in the same community would have acted under the same or similar circumstance, (3) that such failure of breach was the direct cause of the patient's injuries, and (4) that damages to the patient resulted therefrom.*[3]

Direct cause implies that any damage or injuries that resulted from the physician's breach of duty were directly related to that breach and that no intermittent circumstances or intervening acts could have caused the damages.

Damages refers to the injuries suffered by the client. The most common in medical professional liability cases is compensatory damage, which may be general or special.

Compensation for general damages is payment for injuries or losses that are natural or necessary consequences of the physician's neglect (e.g., compensation for pain and suffering or loss of bodily members). Losses must be proved; monetary loss need not be proved.

Special compensation is payment for injuries or losses not necessarily an immediate consequence of the physician's neglect (e.g., cost of remedial medical and hospital care or loss of earnings). Both injuries or losses and monetary value must be proved.[4]

Res Ipsa Loquitur

The doctrine of *res ipsa loquitur*, "the thing speaks for itself," is a rule of law of negligence. It relates chiefly to cases of foreign bodies and slipping instruments in surgical procedures, burns from heating modalities, and injury to a portion of the client's body outside the field of treatment. In other words, the negligence is obvious; the result was such that it could not have occurred without someone being negligent.

Intentional Torts

Intentional torts are intentional acts violating another person's rights or property. The ethical obligation to "do no harm" to a client (nonmalfeasance) is the basis for any intentional tort action. If the principle of nonmalfeasance were never violated and there was no harm to the client there could be no grounds for lawsuits based on intentional torts.

Some of the more common intentional torts likely to occur in ambulatory health care are assault and battery, **defamation,** and invasion of privacy. *Assault* and *battery* are terms often used together; however, assault rarely occurs in the medical setting. Some intentional torts such as assault and battery may also violate criminal laws and may become complaints in both criminal court and civil court. In this situation there will be separate trials, one civil and one criminal. Recall from Chapter 4 that in a civil case the plaintiff must show, by a preponderance of evidence, that a tort has been committed, whereas in a criminal case the prosecution must prove its case beyond a reasonable doubt.

Battery is the unlawful touching, beating, or laying hold of persons or their clothing without consent. When a battery occurs, an individual's right has been invaded. Individuals have the right to be free from invasion of their persons. Regardless of whether the procedure constituting the battery improves the client's health, the client must consent to the touching.

Battery: An Example

A medical assistant, irritated and angered by the client's rudeness and unwillingness to cooperate, gives an injection to the client as ordered by the physician. However, she intentionally twists the needle for the purpose of inflicting pain. Such an action can be called battery.

Defamation is spoken or written words that tend to injure a person's reputation and for which damages can be recovered. One type of defamation is libel, which is false, malicious, defamatory writing, such as published material, effigies, and pictures. Another type of defamation is slander, which is the false and malicious defamatory spoken word. For defamation to be a tort, a third person must hear or see the slander or libel and understand it.

Invasion of privacy is the unauthorized publicity of client information. Medical records and treatments cannot be released without the client's knowledge and permission. Clients have the right to be left alone and the right to be free from unwanted publicity and exposure to public view.

Defamation: An Example

An example of defamation occurs in Vignette 14, in which the secretary makes a potentially derogatory statement: "He must not be licensed to practice."

Invasion of Privacy: Two Examples

An instructor shows photographs of a client's unusual disease or condition to a class without permission.

An ambulatory health care employee permits part of a medical record of a 55-year-old client who gave birth to triplets to be published by the local newspaper without authorization because "it is so unusual."

Torts can be prevented by practicing legally and ethically. The standard of care in an ambulatory health care setting needs to be excellent. The privacy of clients must be guarded, their bodies and possessions must be respected, and their reputations must be protected. The rights of clients are to be protected by all who come in contact with them.

◼◼◼ DOCTRINE OF *RESPONDEAT SUPERIOR*

Professional liability exists for both employer and employee. Physicians are responsible not only for their own actions of negligence but also for the negligent actions of their employees under the doctrine of *respondeat superior.* This Latin phrase means "Let the master answer." Consider the case of a physician assistant (PA) who administers an allergy shot, dismisses the client, and hastens on to the next task without keeping the client under observation for 20 minutes. The client collapses in the parking lot a few minutes later as a result of anaphylactic shock from the injection. The physician employer is responsible for the negligence of the PA. The PA is also liable, and both can be sued.

The physician is responsible for ensuring that all employees perform only those tasks within the scope of their knowledge and training. However, the employer's responsibility does not diminish employees' responsibility to perform only acts within the scope of their knowledge and training. For example, Vignette 3 describes an ambulatory health care employee with only nurse's aid training who assumes a role outside the scope of her practice when she treats the client's wound 12 of 17 times without physician supervision. In this particular case, both the physician and the employee can be found liable if injury occurs to the client as a result of the employee's actions.

The physician's employee has a responsibility to question an order if there is good reason, and a prudent employee in such a position would do so. If the order is not questioned and negligence occurs as a result, both the physician and the employee may be liable.

Professional liability is a concern of all allied health professionals, but physicians are most concerned because they are in a position of higher authority and responsibility.

■■■■ STATUTE OF LIMITATIONS

State legislatures have established statutes of limitations that restrict the time allowed for individuals to initiate any type of legal action. The length of time allowed for starting a lawsuit varies greatly from state to state, generally ranging from 1 to 6 years depending on the severity of the offense.

The statute of limitations most commonly begins at the time when the negligent act was allegedly committed; when the patient discovered or should have discovered the alleged negligence; or when the care, treatment, or client-physician relationship ended. However, states differ in their statute of limitations. Health care professionals should understand state law on the subject, as well as how the law has been interpreted in case law. Tort actions and contracts usually have separate statutes of limitations. The statute of limitations is typically longer for contracts than for torts.

Circumstances that may alter the statute of limitations occur with a person who is legally insane or has not yet reached the age of maturity. Therefore a person declared legally insane will not come under the statute of limitations until the period of insanity has ended. In the case of minors, the period in the statute may not apply until the child has reached the age of maturing, usually 18. This fact is of special concern to pediatricians and obstetricians.

Physicians and their employees must concern themselves with the statute of limitations when considering the retention of their medical records, as well as when they could be involved in a malpractice suit. Legal counsel should be sought for interpretations and advice (Table 5–1).

■■■■ PROFESSIONAL LIABILITY OR MALPRACTICE INSURANCE

The need for physicians to carry professional liability insurance is obvious for numerous reasons. The most important, perhaps, is financial protection. A physician "**going bare**," without insurance, may have to pay any court costs, damages, and attorney fees personally if a malpractice suit is lost.

TABLE 5–1
Statutes of Limitations for Medical Claims Injuries by State

State	Act*	Discov	Accrual*	State	Act*	Discov	Accrual*
Alabama	2/4	6 months		Montana	3/5	3	
Alaska	2	2		Nebraska	2/10	1	
Arizona	2			Nevada	4	2	
Arkansas	2			New Hampshire	3	3	
California	3/3	1		New Jersey			2
Colorado	3		2	New Mexico	3		
Connecticut	2/3	2		New York	2/2		
Delaware	2	3		North Carolina	4	1	
Wash, D.C.			3	North Dakota	6	2	
Florida	2/4	2		Ohio	4		1
Georgia	2/5			Oklahoma		2	
Hawaii	6	2		Oregon	5	2	
Idaho	2			Pennsylvania	2		
Illinois	4	2		Rhode Island	3	3	
Indiana	2			South Carolina	6	3	
Iowa	6	2		South Dakota	2		
Kansas	2/4	2		Tennessee	3	1	
Kentucky	5	1		Texas†	2		
Louisiana	1/3	1		Utah	4	2	
Maine	3			Vermont	3/7	3/2	
Maryland	5	3		Virginia	10	1	2/10
Massachusetts	7		3	Washington	3/8	1	
Michigan	2	6 months		West Virginia	2/10	2	
Minnesota	2			Wisconsin	3/5	1	
Mississippi		2		Wyoming	2	2	
Missouri	2/10						

*Two figures in column indicate the period of time in which to file from act or accrual and the total period in which any claim must be filed. In some states time runs from last date of treatment.
†The Texas statute was held unconstitutional.

Physicians need liability insurance protection whether they are employees or employers. For example, employment in a corporation, a health maintenance organization, or a hospital does not guarantee professional liability coverage. Many employers or institutions carry professional liability insurance merely on themselves or the institution, not on their employees. In some cases, clients sue both the employer and the employee. If employees are covered by an employer's liability policy, they should be specifically named. Employees ought to carry their own professional liability insurance. For example, medical assistants who are members of the American Association of Medical Assistants may purchase professional and personal liability insurance through the organization.

As employers, physicians need professional liability insurance mainly because of the doctrine of *respondeat superior*. Physicians may not be directly negligent, but they are liable for the acts of their employees.

Some physicians are limiting their practice and their professional liability insurance coverage because of the high cost of premiums. For example, a family practitioner may choose not to perform surgeries, thus reducing the cost of professional liability insurance.

Another reason for carrying professional liability insurance is that the physician may be asked for medical advice or assistance from friends or neighbors in a "casual situation." For example, at an outdoor barbecue, a neighbor may ask the physician, "I have this pain in my lower back. What should I do?" In the case of strangers, medical care may be emergent, and the physician may be the only one available to provide the care. An employer's or institution's policy probably will not cover the physician in these situations. The Good Samaritan Law, which may be applied to these situations, will be discussed later.

The kind and amount of liability coverage a physician has varies according to the type of practice, the community economic level, the level of risk of the specialty, and the claims-consciousness of the clients. Most professional liability policies, however, should address (1) what the insurer will pay, (2) effective policy dates, (3) the power of the insurer in obtaining legal counsel, (4) the power of the insurer in seeking settlement, (5) what costs are covered, and (6) how payment is to be made. The policy will specify monetary limits for each claim. For example, a policy may have professional medical liability of 1 million dollars for each claim and 3 million dollars aggregate as a total amount.

The cost of liability insurance is extremely high, ranging from $7,500 to $65,000 per year for a physician.[5] In the 1970s, when malpractice litigation was at its peak, many major insurance carriers stopped offering the coverage. Many of the remaining carriers increased their premiums to survive.

Physicians found it difficult to pay the high premiums, and many sought other professional liability insurance. In some states, physicians banded together to form their own companies to offer lower premiums.

Medical societies have formed insurance companies. Major insurance carriers have also been working with the state medical societies to offer adequate coverage at lower premiums.

Some physicians choose to purchase professional liability insurance for an amount less than advised or to change their practice to be within the coverage of insurance that can be afforded. Whatever liability insurance is purchased, its need has not diminished. In fact, most practices spend 5 to 8 percent of their revenue on malpractice coverage.[6]

ALTERNATIVES TO LITIGATION

Some physicians and institutions have tried solving the malpractice dilemma by alternative dispute resolution (ADR) methods such as arbitration and mediation. These methods eliminate the use of the court system. The client voluntarily agrees, sometimes in advance, with the physician or institution to permit a neutral person or persons to arbitrate the case. The parties involved generally select the impartial third party, who is an expert in the area of controversy. In most instances, the decision of the arbitrator is binding, and there is limited judicial review of the process. In mediation, there is no third party; rather, the mediator is selected by both parties and attempts to facilitate negotiation between them.

A number of states have statutes addressing the use of arbitration and mediation. Some states have established centers for such alternatives to litigation. Generally, the cost of arbitration and mediation is less and will save time for both parties. The case, too, may remain more private.

MALPRACTICE PREVENTION

Generally, if a healthy client-physician relationship exists, malpractice suits are not likely to occur. Some helpful guidelines to prevent malpractice include the following:

1. Perform within the scope of training and education, and do not give advice.
2. Comply with state and federal regulations and statutes.
3. Keep the office safe and equipment in readiness.
4. Practice universal precautions.
5. Log telephone calls. Return all calls to clients within a reasonable time.
6. Avoid treating via the phone.
7. Put verbal instructions in writing, and give a copy to the client.
8. Do not criticize other practitioners.

9. Be sure all diagnostic test results are seen and initialed by the physician before filing.
10. Explain any appointment delays. Do not keep clients waiting for appointments for more than 20 minutes.
11. Select employees carefully, and encourage a team approach.
12. Keep all matters relating to client care confidential.
13. Discuss fees before treatment.
14. Have employees follow up on missed or canceled appointments and document.
15. Treat all persons equally.
16. Never guarantee a cure.
17. Continue to grow professionally.
18. Secure informed consent as much as possible.
19. Listen to clients, and always tell the physician when there is a complaint.
20. Formally document (1) withdrawing from a case and (2) discharging a client.
21. Keep accurate records.
22. Limit practice to scope of training and to a manageable number of clients.
23. Call clients at home the day after outpatient surgery to see how they are doing. Document the follow-up in the client's chart.
24. Chart when clients are called with test results.
25. Chart all canceled appointments and no-shows.
26. Always retain original records or radiographs.
27. Have physician review files before sending accounts to collection.
28. Tell clients how to get care on nights and weekends.
29. Help your physician employer turn your reception area into an education area.
30. Increase your computer literacy. The future of medicine will increasingly use computer technology.
31. Regularly survey clients for satisfaction, and follow suggestions for improvement.

▐▬▬ SUMMARY

Much additional information could be added to the topics in this chapter. The data included should be sufficient to assist physicians and ambulatory health care employees to understand litigation. If office litigation becomes a reality, however, seek professional legal advice promptly.

Employees ought to maintain a **tickler file** of all important dates to recall. These include due dates for license renewals, insurance premiums, and narcotics registrations. Established patterns must be maintained for drug inventory and record keeping. Detailed descriptions and examples of such activities in the office's procedure manual are most helpful.

REFERENCES

1. US Medical Licensure Statistics and Current Licensure Requirements. American Medical Association, Chicago, 1996, p 11.
2. Division of Professional Licensing: The Law Relating to the Practice of Medicine. Department of Licensing, Olympia, Wash, 1987, pp 153–154.
3. Kinn, ME, and Derge, E: The Medical Assistant Administrative and Clinical, ed 7. WB Saunders, Philadelphia, 1993, p 55.
4. Ibid, p 55.
5. Gipe, BT: Tort reform. Cost and Quality Quarterly Journal 1(4):1, 1995.
6. Ibid.

BIBLIOGRAPHY

Aiken, TD, and Catalano, JT: Legal, Ethical and Political Issues in Nursing. FA Davis, Philadelphia, 1994.
Compendium of Selected State Laws Governing Medical Injury Claims. AHCPR Publication Number 93-0053. US Department of Health and Human Services, Rockville, Md, 1993.
Cowdrey, ML, and Drew, M: Basic Law for the Allied Health Professions. Jones & Bartlett, Boston, 1995.
Furrow, BR, et al: Health Law, Vol. 1. West, St Paul, Minn, 1995.
Risk Management Principles and Commentaries for the Medical Office. American Medical Association/Speciality Society Medical Liability Project, Chicago, 1990.

Discussion Questions

1. *For each area of liability discussed in this chapter, give an example that might occur in ambulatory health care.*
2. *Contrast and compare a tort and a breach of contract. Give an example of each.*
3. *Cite two examples of torts an ambulatory health care employee could commit.*
4. *When interviewing for a medical office job that bears much responsibility, you learn that the office professional liability insurance does not cover employees. What options are open to you?*
5. *Generally, one of three situations will determine when the statute of limitations begins. Identify them.*
6. *What might constitute license revocation?*

Public Duties

LEARNING OBJECTIVES

Upon successful completion of this chapter, you will be able to:

1. List seven areas of public duties for physicians.
2. Discuss, in your own words, the importance of filling out birth and death certificates.
3. Identify three circumstances in which a county coroner or medical examiner would be called to investigate a death.
4. Discuss the importance of prompt reporting of death of clients.
5. Describe the process necessary for reporting communicable and notifiable diseases.
6. Restate the protocol to use for reporting adverse events to vaccines and toxoids.
7. List at least four injuries that are reportable.
8. Discuss elder and child abuse laws.
9. Identify four types of professionals who are required to report suspected child abuse.
10. Describe the process used in gathering and securing evidence in the ambulatory health care setting.
11. Explain, in your own words, the drug abuse problem.
12. List four possible ways to prevent drug abuse in ambulatory health care.
13. Define the Good Samaritan Law.

DEFINITIONS

Autopsy. Examination by specially trained medical personnel of the body after death to determine cause of death or pathologic conditions.
Coroner. An official, usually elected, who investigates death from sudden, unknown, or violent causes; may or may not be a physician.
Fiduciary. A trustee relationship between individuals.

Notifiable or reportable disease. A disease that concerns the public welfare and requires reporting to the proper authority; a potentially pathologic condition that may be transmitted directly or indirectly from one individual to another.

Notifiable or reportable injury. An injury that concerns the public welfare and requires reporting to the proper authority; for example, injuries resulting from gun or knife wounds.

Some details of many duties of physicians will become the responsibility of ambulatory health care employees. Physicians, as licensed professionals, have statutory and regulatory requirements they must follow. Reports of births; stillbirths; deaths; communicable diseases; specific injuries; and child, elder, and drug abuse are a few examples. Reporting requirements vary among states. To become familiar with your particular state's reporting requirements, refer to the state's statutes and administrative regulations, which are available in most county libraries. Colleges have access to law books, especially those specific to statutes. Reference librarians can offer valuable help in locating the appropriate statute. In addition, ambulatory health care employees should contact the local and state medical societies. Most medical societies have an attorney "on call" who can offer practical guidance. Contact your local health department and local law enforcement for reporting forms and information. Both agencies may be willing to send written information. Visits to the local health department may be useful.

Good Samaritan Laws are included in this chapter so that physicians and their staff members realize that their professional responsibility goes beyond the ambulatory health care setting.

Gathering and reporting statistical data and information may become an impersonal task, but physicians and their staffs need to remember that these data represent individuals. Therefore the task is a personal matter. Deaths, rapes, and abuse are sensitive issues. Individuals involved need special care.

Consider your responsibilities if the following circumstances occurred in your office:

1. A young husband, grieving his wife's sudden death, is told that cause of death is still undetermined pending laboratory results.
2. A 68-year-old widow is seen today by your physician after a sexual assault.
3. The owner of a local restaurant has just tested positive for infectious hepatitis. He cannot return to work during the infectious period.

If the physicians office has established policies regarding these matters, the inquiry and reporting processes will be facilitated, and the special care often required of these clients will be encouraged. Each employee should know what kind of inquiry to make, how reporting is done, who is responsible, what information is required, and when and where the report is filed. A copy should always be kept for the office. Be aware of any community agencies that are available to provide information for the office and to provide valuable services for the clients.

■■■■ BIRTHS AND DEATHS

The recording of births and deaths is an important function of the physician. These certificates are legal documents and require truthfulness and prompt and proper completion. In some states, a criminal penalty will result if birth or death certificates are not properly completed. Some states refuse to accept certificates completed in inks other than black; others refuse to accept a certificate with any blanks.

> A birth certificate will be used throughout a person's life to prove age, parentage, and citizenship. For example, a child will need a birth certificate when entering school. Adults will require a birth certificate to register to vote or to obtain a driver's license, a marriage license, a passport, veteran's benefits, welfare aid, and social security benefits.

Certificate requirements vary from state to state. A stillbirth or fetal death, in which the fetus has not reached the 20th week of gestation, may require neither a birth nor a death certificate. In some states, however, a special stillbirth form is used; in others, it is necessary to file both a birth and death certificate. If the birth is considered a live birth and then the infant dies, both a standard birth and death certificate need to be completed.

In the event of a nonhospital birth, the person in attendance is responsible for initiating the birth certificate. In such a delivery, a parent should verify that the process is completed according to state regulations.

Check with your state's health or vital statistics department, which offers information regarding reporting of birth and death certificates. This agency provides detailed information for completing the standard forms. Figure 6–1 is an example of the standard certificate of birth. Figure 6–2 is an example of the standard certificate of death.

Generally speaking, physicians sign a certificate giving the cause of death of the deceased upon whom they have been in professional attendance. Otherwise, someone of greater authority, such as the county health officer or **coroner,** will assume the responsibility. In some states, a physician is for-

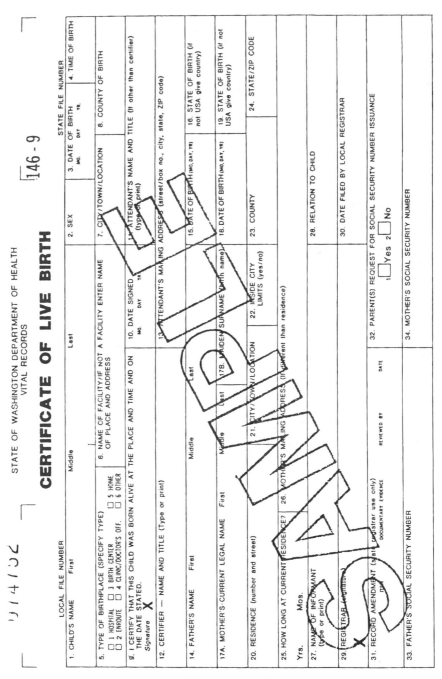

Figure 6–1. Birth certificate.

FATHER

35. OF HISPANIC ORIGIN OR DESCENT? (Ancestry) (Specify yes or no) If yes, specify Cuban, Mexican, Puerto Rican, etc. □1 Yes □2 No

36. RACE (White, Black, Asian or Pacific Islander, American Indian, Hispanic, etc.) (Specify)

37. OCCUPATION (Indicate most recent employment) (pressman, painter, computer programmer) (Specify)

38. TYPE OF BUSINESS OR INDUSTRY (paper mill, hwy. construction, nuclear) (Specify)

MOTHER

39. OF HISPANIC ORIGIN OR DESCENT? (Ancestry) (Specify yes or no) If yes, specify Cuban, Mexican, Puerto Rican, etc. □1 Yes □2 No

40. RACE (White, Black, Asian or Pacific Islander, American Indian, Hispanic, etc.) (Specify)

41. OCCUPATION (Indicate most recent employment) (fruit packer, cashier, registered nurse) (Specify)

42. TYPE OF BUSINESS OR INDUSTRY (apple orchard, retail sales, hospital) (Specify)

CHILD

43. OF HISPANIC ORIGIN OR DESCENT? (Ancestry) (Specify yes or no) If yes, specify Cuban, Mexican, Puerto Rican, etc. □1 Yes □2 No

44. RACE (White, Black, Asian or Pacific Islander, American Indian, Hispanic, etc.) (Specify)

PARENTAL IDENTIFICATION OF CHILD'S ETHNICITY AND RACE. (Items 43 and 44)

45. PRIOR LIVE BIRTHS (Do not include this birth)
□ NONE NOW LIVING | NOW DEAD
NUMBER ____ | ____
DATE LAST LIVE BIRTH (MO. YR)

46. OTHER PREGNANCY OUTCOMES (Not live births)
□ NONE
20 WKS OR MORE
LESS THAN 20 WKS
DATE LAST SPONTANEOUS OUTCOME
NUMBER SPONTANEOUS ____
NUMBER INDUCED (Any gest., age) ____
DATE LAST INDUCED

47. TOTAL PRIOR PREGNANCIES

48. DATE LAST NORMAL MENSES BEGAN (MO. DAY YR.)

49. IS MOTHER MARRIED? □1 YES □2 NO

50. MONTH OF PREGNANCY PRENATAL CARE BEGAN (1st, 2nd, 3rd, etc.)

51. TOTAL NUMBER OF PRENATAL VISITS (If none, enter 0)

52. CLINICAL ESTIMATE OF GESTATION (WEEKS)

53. MOTHER TRANSFERRED AFTER ATTEMPTED DELIVERY? □1 Yes □2 No
If yes, from ____ Birth Ctr. ____ Home ____ Other

54. PLURALITY—Single, Twin, Triplet, etc. (Specify)

55. IF NOT SINGLE BIRTH—born 1st, 2nd, 3rd, etc. (Specify)

56. BIRTH WEIGHT lbs. ____ ozs. ____ or ____ grams

57. APGAR SCORE 1 Min. ____ 5 Min. ____

58. INFANT TRANSFERRED TO ANOTHER FACILITY? □1 Yes □2 No □3 Unk.

Figure 6–1. (continued)

CHECK ALL BOX(ES) IN EACH COLUMN THAT APPLY OR WRITE IN "OTHER" IF NO BOXES APPLY

59. MEDICAL RISK FACTORS FOR THIS PREGNANCY
1. Anemia (Hct.<30/Hgb.<10)
2. Cardiac disease
3. Acute or chronic lung disease
4. Diabetes, Gest.☐ Estab.☐
5. Genital herpes—active ☐ HX ☐
6. Polyhydramnios
7. Oligohydramnios
8. Hemoglobinopathy
9. Hypertension, chronic
10. Hypertension, pregnancy-associated
11. Eclampsia
12. Incompetent cervix
13. Previous infant 4000 + grams
14. Previous preterm or small-for-gestational age infant
15. Renal disease
16. Rh sensitization
17. 1st trimester bleeding
18. Epilepsy
19. Syphilis
20. Rubella—test positive
21. None
22. Other (specify)

60. OTHER RISK FACTORS FOR THIS PREGNANCY
1. Tobacco use during pregnancy?
☐ Yes ☐ No   Av. No. cig. per day____
2. Alcohol use during pregnancy?
☐ Yes ☐ No   Av. No. drinks per wk____
3. Weight gained during preg.____lbs.

61. OBSTETRIC PROCEDURES
1. Amniocentesis
If yes, specify trimesters ☐1 ☐2 ☐3
2. Electronic fetal monitoring
3. Induction of labor
4. Stimulation of labor
5. Tocolysis
6. Ultrasound
7. None
8. Other (specify)

62. METHOD OF DELIVERY
1. Vaginal
2. Vaginal birth after previous C-section
3. Primary C-section
4. Repeat C-section with no labor
5. Repeat C-section with trial of labor
6. Forceps
7. Vacuum extraction
8. Other (specify)

63. COMPLICATIONS OF LABOR AND/OR DELIVERY
1. Febrile (> 100°F or 38°C)
2. Meconium, moderate/heavy
3. Premature rupture of membrane (>12 hrs)
4. Abruptio placenta
5. Placenta previa
6. Other excessive bleeding
7. Seizures during labor
8. Precipitous labor (<3 hrs)
9. Prolonged labor (>20 hrs)
10. Dysfunctional labor
11. Breech/Malpresentation
12. Cephalopelvic disproportion
13. Cord prolapse
14. Anesthetic complications
15. Fetal distress
16. None
17. Other (specify)

64. ABNORMAL CONDITIONS OF THE NEWBORN
1. Anemia (Hct<39/Hgb.<13)
2. Birth injury
3. Fetal alcohol syndrome
4. Hyaline membrane disease/RDS
5. Meconium aspiration syndrome
6. Drug withdrawal syndrome in newborn
7. Assisted ventilation <30 min.
8. Assisted ventilation ≥30 min.
9. Seizures
Continued Next Column

64. ABNORMAL CONDITIONS OF THE NEWBORN (CONTINUED)
10. Sepsis
11. Asphyxia/Depression
12. Erb's palsy
13. Jaundice (greater than 10 in 1st 48 hrs.)
14. None
15. Other (specify)

65. CONGENITAL ANOMALIES OF CHILD
1. Anencephalus
2. Spina bifida/Meningocele
3. Hydrocephalus
4. Microcephalus
5. Other central nervous system anomalies (specify)
6. Heart malformations
7. Other circulatory/respiratory anomalies (specify)
8. Rectal atresia/stenosis
9. Tracheo-esophageal fistula/Esophageal atresia
10. Omphalocele/Gastroschisis
11. Other gastrointestinal anomalies (specify)
12. Malformed genitalia
13. Renal agenesis
14. Other urogenital anomalies (specify)
15. Cleft lip/palate
16. Polydactyly/Syndactyly/Adactyly
17. Club foot
18. Diaphragmatic hernia
19. Other musculoskeletal/integumental anomalies (specify)
20. Down's syndrome
21. Other chromosomal anomalies (specify)
22. None
23. Other anomalies (specify)

FOR SPECIFIC ITEM INSTRUCTIONS SEE HANDBOOK

DOH 110-012 1/90 - 1419-

Figure 6-1. *(continued)*

bidden by law to sign certain death certificates. Examples include a death caused by criminal activity, a death without a physician present, a death from an undetermined cause, or a violent or unlawful death. These cases are immediately turned over to a coroner, medical examiner, or equivalent official for investigation and issuance of a death certificate. A death may also need to be reported to the coroner in the following instances: a death occurring within 24 hours after a client is admitted to a hospital or licensed health care facility, nonattendance by a physician during the 3 days before death, or death of an individual outside a hospital or licensed health care facility. The physician should not send the remains to a mortician without authorization from the next of kin or other person responsible for funeral expenses.

Prompt reporting by the physician is required so that the remains will not be disturbed and evidence will not be lost. This is particularly significant if an investigation or **autopsy** is to be performed. The physician may be the only one who knows the client's current medical history and treatment. As such, when called to the death scene, the physician may discover facts inconsistent with the client's medical history and can then notify the authorities. Law enforcement may begin an investigation resulting in prosecution of criminals and alteration of survivors' rights or other benefits. Also, if the death is the result of an accident or an occupational or environmental hazard, an autopsy or investigation may identify the actual cause of death. Thus the physician is a key individual in the discovery of facts surrounding death, and prompt reporting is essential.

As a courtesy to the family, it is imperative that the death certificate be completed and signed as quickly as possible so that funeral and financial arrangements can begin. Many states have a requirement that the death certificate be filed within 24 to 72 hours. The physician's office staff should realize that no arrangements can be made until the death certificate is signed.

> The death certificate proves a person has died. A certified copy of a death certificate is useful in obtaining access to insurance policy monies, bank accounts, safe-deposit boxes, dispersal of estates, real property transactions, tax base information, Internal Revenue Service information, and veteran's benefits.

COMMUNICABLE AND NOTIFIABLE DISEASES

A disease is reportable (**notifiable or reportable disease**) when it concerns the public welfare and when it is a potentially pathologic condition that may be transmitted directly or indirectly from one individual to another. The reporting of communicable diseases varies among states; however,

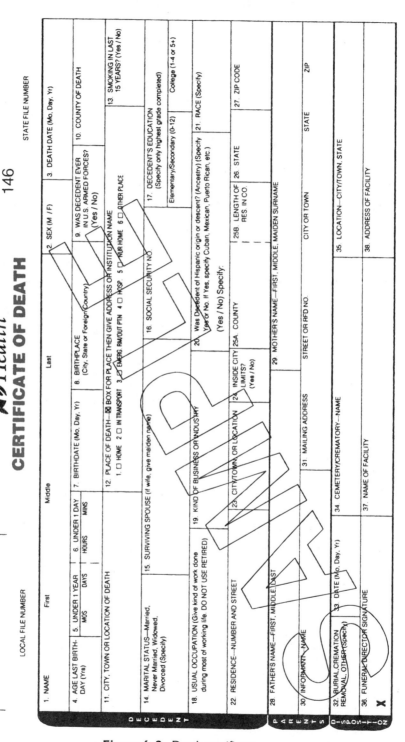

Figure 6–2. Death certificate.

TO BE COMPLETED ONLY BY **CERTIFYING PHYSICIAN**

TO BE COMPLETED ONLY BY **MEDICAL EXAMINER OR CORONER**

39 **TO THE BEST OF MY KNOWLEDGE**, DEATH OCCURRED AT THE TIME, DATE AND PLACE AND WAS DUE TO THE CAUSE(S) STATED.

SIGNATURE AND TITLE

X

43 ON THE BASIS OF EXAMINATION AND/OR INVESTIGATION, IN MY OPINION DEATH OCCURRED AT THE TIME, DATE AND PLACE AND WAS DUE TO THE CAUSE(S) STATED

SIGNATURE AND TITLE

X

40. DATE SIGNED (Mo., Day, Yr)

41 HOUR OF DEATH (24 Hrs)

44 DATE SIGNED (Mo., Day, Yr)

45 HOUR OF DEATH (24 Hrs)

42 NAME AND TITLE OF ATTENDING PHYSICIAN IF OTHER THAN CERTIFIER (Type or Print)

46 PRONOUNCED DEAD (Mo., Day, Yr)

47 HOUR PRONOUNCED DEAD (24 Hrs.)

48 NAME AND ADDRESS OF CERTIFIER—PHYSICIAN, MEDICAL EXAMINER OR CORONER (Type or Print)

49 ME/CORONER FILE NUMBER

50. ENTER THE DISEASES, INJURIES, OR COMPLICATIONS WHICH CAUSED THE DEATH:

IMMEDIATE CAUSE (Final disease or condition resulting in death).

A.

DUE TO, OR AS A CONSEQUENCE OF:

INTERVAL BETWEEN ONSET AND DEATH

DO NOT ENTER THE MODE OF DYING, SUCH AS CARDIAC OR RESPIRATORY ARREST, SHOCK, OR HEART FAILURE. LIST ONLY ONE CAUSE ON EACH LINE.

B

DUE TO, OR AS A CONSEQUENCE OF:

INTERVAL BETWEEN ONSET AND DEATH

Sequentially list conditions, if any, leading to immediate cause. Enter UNDERLYING CAUSE (Disease or injury which initiated events resulting in death) LAST.

C.

DUE TO, OR AS A CONSEQUENCE OF:

INTERVAL BETWEEN ONSET AND DEATH

D.

INTERVAL BETWEEN ONSET AND DEATH

51. OTHER SIGNIFICANT CONDITIONS—CONDITIONS CONTRIBUTING TO DEATH BUT NOT RESULTING IN THE UNDERLYING CAUSE GIVEN ABOVE:

52. AUTOPSY? (Yes / No)

53 WAS CASE REFERRED TO MEDICAL EXAMINER OR CORONER? (Yes / No)

54 ACC. SUICIDE. HOM., UNDET., OR PENDING INVEST. (Specify)

55 INJURY DATE (Mo, Day, Yr)

56 HOUR OF INJURY (24 Hrs)

57 DESCRIBE HOW INJURY OCCURRED:

58 INJURY AT WORK? (Yes / No)

59 PLACE OF INJURY—AT HOME, FARM, STREET, FACTORY, OFFICE BLDG., ETC. (Specify)

60 LOCATION—STREET OR RFD NO., CITY/TOWN, STATE

61 RECORD AMENDMENT (Registrar use only)
ITEM   DOCUMENTARY EVIDENCE   REVIEWED BY   DATE

62 REGISTRAR SIGNATURE

X

63 DATE RECEIVED (Mo., Day, Yr.)

FOR INSTRUCTIONS SEE BACK AND HANDBOOK

DOH 110-008 (Rev. 7/91) (formerly DSHS 9-150)

Figure 6–2. *(continued)*

local health departments publish and periodically update lists of 30 or more notifiable diseases and the required reporting format.

Physicians have the duty to report notifiable diseases by phone, by mail, or electronically. Reports are usually made by the office assistant, who telephones the county health department and furnishes the following information:

1. Disease (or suspected disease)
2. Name, address, age, and occupation of person with suspected disease
3. Date of onset of disease
4. Name of person reporting

To report by mail, use the appropriate case report cards furnished by the health department. Many diseases are reported on special forms. A check with your local health department may reveal 20 or more specific forms for diseases. Some states encourage reporting by phone, with the statistical data being collected by the health department. Other states require that the initial paperwork be completed at the time the notifiable disease is detected. Whatever method of reporting is used, be prompt, consistent, factual, and complete. Keep a copy of the report for the office files. The health department will attempt to determine the source of infection and mode of transmission so that public health will be protected.

All health care providers who administer certain childhood vaccines and toxoids are required by law to record certain information and report adverse events. In 1986 Congress passed the National Childhood Vaccine Injury Act listing the following vaccines and toxoids:

Diphtheria and tetanus toxoids and pertussis vaccine
Pertussis vaccine
Measles, mumps, and rubella
Poliovirus vaccine live, oral
Poliovirus vaccine inactivated

The information to be recorded includes the date of the vaccine's administration; the manufacturer and lot number of the vaccine; and the name, address, and title of the person administering the vaccine. Any adverse events after administration would also be recorded. Many pediatric offices require signed informed consent forms before administration of vaccines and are offering written information to parents and guardians about vaccines and toxoids. The same requirements may apply to influenzae and hepatitis B vaccines.

For more detailed information, consult your health department or the following two references: *Report of the Committee on Infectious Disease,* American Academy of Pediatrics, PO Box 1034, Evanston, IL 60204; and *Control of Communicable Disease in Man,* The American Public Health Association, 1015 Eighteenth Street, NW, Washington, DC 20036.

Vignette 7

A patient underwent elective surgery for total hip replacement. Early during the surgery, the assistant surgeon became so ill he had to lie down on the operating room floor. The hospital called another physician (Dr. Howard), who had his office across the street from the hospital. He canceled his office appointments, came to the hospital, and completed the surgery with the surgeon. After the surgery, the patient suffered complications and sued Dr. Howard.

Outcome: Under the Good Samaritan Law in California, the court ruled that Dr. Howard "did not commit any willful act or omission" while assisting the surgeon. Dr. Howard was rendering emergency care in "good faith," which addresses the quality of the intentions and not the quality of the care delivered. Also, Dr. Howard had no preexisting duty of professional care to this patient; the patient was not an established patient of his. This is another requirement of the Good Samaritan Law.- Further, the court stated that, as a matter of public policy, the Good Samaritan Law encourages physicians to respond to emergency requests. *Perkins v Howard,* 283 Cal Rptr 764 (1991).

Note: Although this case involves physicians working in a hospital, the legal implications are strong for office assistants and office settings as well.

REPORTABLE INJURIES

An injury is reportable (**notifiable or reportable injury**) when it concerns the public welfare and requires reporting to the proper authority, for example, injuries resulting from gun or knife wounds. Some states have detailed requirements for reporting injuries. Others have none. Check with the local and state medical associations and law enforcement agencies for specific information.

Generally, injuries caused by lethal weapons, such as guns and knives, are reported, and persons are treated in emergency or hospital facilities. When rape victims or battered persons seek treatment from private physicians, they may be treated in the office or immediately referred to the emergency room of a local hospital.

Questions may arise concerning reporting requirements. For example, if an adult rape victim reports for medical care in the office after an assault, must the assault be reported? If the physician suspects elder or spousal abuse, must it be reported?

At least 50 state variances govern the reporting of such incidents. In some states, marital rape laws may mandate reporting of spousal abuse. In these states, failure to report elder and spousal abuse may specifically be considered a misdemeanor.

Basic considerations when dealing with the assault victim include the following:

1. Consider the victim's vulnerability to future assault.
2. Respect the victim's right not to report abuse if this is permissible by law.
3. Acquaint yourself with your community's resources, and refer the victim when appropriate.
4. Remember that both the victim and the abuser need professional care and have rights protected by law.

Urban areas have community service agencies such as Rape Relief and sexual assault centers. The physician may refer the victim to such an agency for additional, specialized services. However, if these services are unavailable or the victim chooses to be treated by the physician alone, the physician needs information from law enforcement agencies regarding reporting the incident and obtaining, securing, and handling medicolegal evidence.

The victim should be treated as soon as possible after the injury or assault, not only for the victim's welfare but also to preserve evidence of possible criminal acts. Rape victims, in particular, need to feel supported and cared for and to feel that the violent act will make no difference in how they are treated by people.

ELDER ABUSE

The majority of states have enacted legislation addressing elder abuse, which is abuse of persons 60 years and older. The laws generally name a health care professional as one who reports the abuse, and in some states, it is a requirement to report suspected elder abuse. States may protect the reporter from civil and criminal liability. The reporting agency varies in each state but generally is a social service or welfare agency. The definition of abuse is generally physical abuse not caused by accident; however, some laws also address **fiduciary**, neglect, and abandonment.

To gain knowledge about your state laws, several avenues are available. Contact your local state legislators and ask for a copy of a specific law, call your legislative hot line and ask for a copy of a state statute, or visit your nearest law library. If your local college has a paralegal program, students may be available to assist you in locating copies of laws. Most libraries have reference librarians who are helpful.

CHILD ABUSE

Child abuse is deplored by everyone. Yet in one day in the life of American children, three die from child abuse, and 30 more are wounded by guns. Health care professionals rush to the aid of an innocent child struck down by serious illness or genetic defect. For example, a staggering 1.5 million dollars was spent over a period of 4 years to save a child born with no gut. After the first liver and bowel transplant failed and the subsequent failure of an experimental transplant of liver, kidney, pancreas, and large and small intestines occurred, and widespread malignancy from side effects of immunosuppression racked the infant's body, life support was finally shut off.

Yet two infants thrown from a third-floor apartment by an angry father gets only a few inches in the local newspaper. No one had the few minutes it takes to find out how to get those two children to safety.

Incidents of child abuse and neglect may be seen in a hospital or a physician's office when a child displays fractures, burns, severe bruises, and questionable injuries. Not so obvious injuries may include dislocations, cerebrospinal trauma, and internal injuries resulting from blows to the abdomen. Malnutrition, lower than expected growth rate, poor hygiene, gross dental problems, and unattended medical needs also may indicate neglect or abuse.

Currently, each state has statutes or laws defining child abuse and mandating that suspected child abuse and neglect be reported. Any person who has reasonable cause to suspect that a child may be the victim of abuse or neglect may report, in good faith, to law enforcement or child protection agencies. Such persons are protected against liability as a result of making the report, provided there is reasonable cause to suspect child abuse or neglect.

Certain individuals are required to report suspected abuse and neglect. These include health professionals, social service personnel, law enforcement personnel, educators, and any professional person working with children. Some states also allow a hospital administrator or a physician to detain a child legally without a guardian's consent in such instances.

The function of reporting is to identify incidents of suspected abuse and neglect, not to prove abuse or neglect. Failure to report suspected abuse or neglect may result in civil or criminal penalties.

The report may be oral, written, or both. Immediate reporting is paramount so that a proper investigation can be initiated. Information required in the report may include the following[1]:

1. Name, address, and age of child
2. Name and address of child's parents (or guardians)
3. Nature and extent of the injury, neglect, or abuse
4. Any evidence of previous incidents of abuse or neglect, including their nature and extent

5. Any other information that may be helpful in establishing the cause of the child's injuries, neglect, or death and the identity of the perpetrator(s)

If a crime has been committed, law enforcement must be notified.

Child abuse and neglect are difficult problems. Although laws were meant to protect the welfare of the child, they may, in fact, safeguard the family unit more. However, physicians and employees need to be advocates of the child's well-being without being judgmental of the parents.

CRITICAL THINKING EXERCISES

Identify cultures in which abuse (child, spousal, adult, elder, drug) is defined differently than in the United States. For example, consider the following:

1. The use of a belt to spank a child
2. A cultural attitude that recommends circumcision of young girls (removal of clitoris and suturing the vaginal opening)
3. A culture in which the use of illegal drugs may result in beheading
4. A culture that severely punishes a rapist and supports financially and emotionally the female victim or a child born of that rape
5. A culture that kills its infants or its infirm if there is not enough food and shelter available
6. Developing countries in which few or no vaccines are available for children

---

EVIDENCE

Gathering of evidence is more likely to occur in the emergency room or hospital setting. There will be situations in the ambulatory health care setting, however, in which employees and physicians need to be knowledgeable of methods of proper collection and preservation of evidence. (See Chapter 4 for an explanation of the trial process.) When in doubt, seek professional guidance from attorneys and the proper authorities.

In the ambulatory health care setting, physicians may gather legal evidence knowingly or unknowingly. Later they may be asked to offer the evidence or will be subpoenaed to give the evidence. Office situations in which evidence will be collected include the female toddler's urinalysis showing sperm, the young boy seeking medical treatment because he has been sexually assaulted, or a client entering with a superficial knife wound. Circumstances just described may involve physicians as witnesses in litigation. Proper examination and documentation are essential.

One of the first ways evidence is documented is through medical records. Malpractice lawsuits are commonly lost because of improper documentation in medical records. Specifically, physicians must record the time of client arrival; a complete explanation of the client's condition, both physical and emotional; and what was done for the client. Obviously, treatment of the client is primary, but documentation in the client's medical record must follow. The written documentation must be clear, concise, complete, and in order.

Evidence may be in the form of a complete written description, roentgenograms, photographs, clothing, samples for laboratory testing, or samples of foreign objects. Roentgenograms and photographs need to be dated and labeled with the client's name. Photographs may need a brief description relating what is pictured. Both roentgenograms and photographs should be stored in envelopes to protect them. Any objects and clothing should be properly and carefully removed, labeled, and stored. Clothing should not be cut unless necessary and then along seams. Do not rinse or wash clothing. In fact, do not handle clothing any more than necessary to avoid changing or damaging evidence. Any body fluids, such as vomitus or gastric washing, should be saved, especially in poisoning cases, for future analysis.

You may be requested by law enforcement to take client samples such as blood; semen; vaginal, oral, or rectal smears; or skin, fingernail, or hair clippings. Samples must be properly labeled and preserved. Every piece of evidence needs to be preserved as much as possible and securely stored in a locked place to avoid tampering or loss.

Having only one employee handle all evidence can prevent it from becoming inadmissible because it cannot be properly traced or verified. When giving evidence to the proper authorities, ask for a receipt for office files. Know to whom you are giving the evidence.

Physicians should cooperate with law enforcement authorities who need to talk to the client. The physician and office staff should not be overprotective of the client, nor should the client be jeopardized. The authorities need to receive information on the client so that they can begin their investigation immediately.

If a client dies in the office or arrives dead, the medical examiner or coroner should be called immediately and the remains should not be touched or removed. Office employees should not touch, tamper, or remove any tubes or paraphernalia from the client. Leave the deceased as is; otherwise, evidence may be useless to authorities.

DRUG ABUSE

Drug misuse or abuse is found in every sector of society. No one is exempt. Drug abuse occurs in affluent communities and in the ghetto. It is commonplace in schools, in colleges, in all the professions, and in industry. Pharmacists receive fake telephone prescription orders. Physicians are pestered by abusers seeking controlled substances for their personal use or for resale in the streets. Health professionals also are vulnerable to drug abuse, perhaps more so because of the availability of drugs to them. Few statutes or regulatory requirements relate to drug abuse other than the Controlled Substances Act discussed in Chapter 4. However, physicians and their employees have a public duty to be alert to this problem and to do everything possible to prevent its increase.

A common problem is a drug abuser securing the same prescription drug from more than one physician and pharmacy in an area. Often abusers go from door to door of medical clinics and offices with a convincing tale of woe or set of symptoms that may warrant a prescription drug. The office assistant often is convinced by the abuser that this is a valid complaint and may be coerced into becoming an advocate for the abuser. Another problem occurs when a physician becomes what is known as a "script doctor," one who freely and excessively prescribes potentially dangerous drugs.

Some communities have established hot lines so that descriptions of suspected drug abusers and their mode of operation can be communicated to physicians and pharmacists in the area. One technique that works well is for the assistant or physician to ask for a picture identification card of each new client. Most abusers will not produce such identification. An assistant should also be advised that the physician will authorize no prescriptions without first seeing the client.

Physicians and office staff must keep prescription pads secure. Controlled substances should not be kept on the premises if at all possible. Any that are kept must be under lock and key and immediately reported if stolen or lost. Be alert to the regular client who may be seeing more than one doctor for the same complaint and receiving several prescriptions. Carefully question clients during examination. Pharmacists watch closely for this problem, but the number of pharmacies in large cities makes effective control nearly impossible.

The market for prescription drugs on the street is a lucrative one. Physicians and health professionals must establish firm and clear office procedures to curb the increase of drug misuse and abuse. A comprehensive substance abuse history should be taken from all clients.

GOOD SAMARITAN LAWS

Good Samaritan statutes exist in all 50 states, yet their content varies widely with regard to who is protected, the standard of care required, and the circumstances under which protection is provided. The statute itself is a legal doctrine meant to encourage physicians and health care professionals to render emergency first aid treatment to accident victims without liability for negligence. It does not apply to an emergency arising in a clinic, hospital, or office where the client-physician relationship exists. However, the scene of emergency may include the emergency room of the hospital in the event of a medical disaster.[2]

The statutes mainly apply to physicians, but many also address other health care professionals. A few statutes include laypersons. In most states, no one, including physicians and health care professionals, has the legal obligation to render first aid in a life-threatening situation. Most Good Samaritan statutes merely attempt to protect the physician or health care professional who does and acts "in good faith" and "without gross negligence." In some states, you must be a Good Samaritan or face a penalty, whereas in others, legislation states that physicians must administer emergency treatment to the best of their ability.

The majority of Good Samaritan statutes are poorly written and leave many unanswered questions. Not many define the following: What is an emergency? What is care rendered gratuitously? Where and to what extent can care be given to be covered by the statute?

Many health care professionals are reluctant to render aid in an emergency. Reasons for this attitude may include the poorly written laws, the legal and professional advice to be cautious, and the fear that the situation may require skills outside of one's training and education. The health care professional may be as anxious to avoid getting involved as the layperson. The risk of liability, however, has been grossly exaggerated. Rarely are lawsuits filed against a Good Samaritan, whether physician or nurse.

All health care professionals and their employees ought to know their Good Samaritan Laws and specifically what and to whom they address. The ethical issue must also be considered. The American Medical Association (AMA), in the Principles of Medical Ethics (see Appendix I), states that physicians should respond to any requests for assistance in an emergency. Certainly, the legal and ethical ramifications of rendering aid in an emergency should be considered before an emergency presents itself. Although the health care professional may feel inadequate and unprotected in an emergency, the general public considers such a professional to be far more qualified than any layperson appearing on the scene.

Health care professionals who do render aid in an emergency must remember to treat within the scope of their training and to give adequate care in light of the circumstances. They also should take comfort in the fact that the chance of a lawsuit is slim.

REFERENCES

1. Washington State Department of Social and Health Services: Protecting the Abused and Neglected Child. Department of Social and Health Services, Olympia, Wash, 1980, pp 22–163.
2. Furrow, BR, et al: Health Law, Vol. 1. West, St. Paul, Minn, 1995, p 388.

BIBLIOGRAPHY

Flight, MR: Good Samaritan Laws. Professional Medical Assistant 23(4):15, 1990.

Hill, JK: Secret lives: Recognizing the signs of addiction. Professional Medical Assistant 27(1):8, 1994.

In brief: One day in the life of American children, Children's Defense Fund, 1994. Hastings Cent Rep 24(1):3, 1994.

McAfee, RE: Violence in America: Making a difference one patient at a time. Professional Medical Assistant 29(1):5, 1996.

Nicholson, RH: Old world news: What's a child worth? Hastings Cent Rep 24(1):5, 1994.

Rice, J: Immunization: The best protection against vaccine preventable diseases. Professional Medical Assistant 27(5):8, 1994.

Vogtsberger, KN: Identifying drug seeking, drug abusing patients. Professional Medical Assistant 29(3):5, 1996.

Discussion Questions

1. *Using the three examples described in the box at the beginning of the chapter, discuss your responsibilities in each situation, the possible referral agencies available, and the possible problems encountered. How can you be of assistance to your physician employer?*

2. *What problems occur when a death certificate remains unsigned?*

3. *What are the future implications if a birth is not reported?*

4. *Explore possible referral agencies in your community, and share your findings.*

5. *The physician gives you an envelope of roentgenograms and a sealed bag of clothing items and asks you to keep them safe until law enforcement officials arrive. How would you keep them safe? Why is this important?*

6. *Describe different drug abusers who may frequent a medical office. How can office personnel be alert to these abusers?*

7. *Under what circumstances might a physician decide not to render emergency aid?*

chapter 7

Consent

LEARNING OBJECTIVES

Upon successful completion of this chapter, you will be able to:

1. Define the term *consent* and explain, in your own words, why consent is important.
2. Give an example of verbal consent, nonverbal consent, and written consent.
3. Compare informed and uninformed consent.
4. List the four elements of the doctrine of informed consent.
5. Identify the following special situations in consent: minors, spouses, language barriers, and when consent is not necessary.
6. Discuss the role of the ambulatory health care employee in obtaining consent.

DEFINITIONS

Consent. The affirmation by a client to allow touching, examination, or treatment by medically authorized personnel.

Doctrine of informed consent. Specific guidelines for consent, usually identified by medical practice acts at the state level. Clients' right to know before agreeing to treatments, care, and procedures. Physicians must use terms or language that clients understand. Clients voluntarily give permission to allow touching, examination, or treatment by medically authorized personnel and understand what their consent means.

Minor. A person who has not reached the age of maturity. The age of maturity is 18 years in most jurisdictions.

1. **Emancipated minor.** A person younger than 18 years of age who is free of parental care and is financially responsible for himself or herself.

2. **Mature minor.** A person, usually younger than 18 years of age, who possesses sufficient understanding and appreciation of the nature and consequences of treatment despite chronologic age.

Uninformed consent. Client gives permission to allow touching, examination, or treatment by medically authorized personnel but does not understand what has been consented to.

All ambulatory health care employees at one time or another will be involved in the **consent** process with the clients they serve. Although the health care provider has the primary responsibility to inform the client of the proposed treatment to obtain consent for a procedure, clients commonly ask questions of ambulatory health care employees. Consequently, everyone must understand all aspects of consent.

▪▬▬ DEFINITION

Consent is the voluntary affirmation by a client to allow touching, examination, or treatment by medically authorized personnel. Consent allows clients to determine what will be done with their bodies. Without consent, intentional touching can be considered a criminal offense. Consent is authorization given by implications of a client's behavior or a medical contract or by law. Consent is obtained through word or action. Consent may be given orally, expressed by nonverbal behavior, or expressed in writing. Some state laws mandate that written consent is necessary for any invasive procedure. Further, some states may find ambulatory health care employees liable for failing to give information to clients. Health care professionals may be legally liable for offering information and for obtaining informed consent from clients. Be aware of your state's **doctrine of informed consent** laws. Consider the following examples:

1. A client calls complaining of a persistent, productive cough. When the receptionist makes the appointment with the physician, the client has given consent for examination, which may include throat examination and culture.

2. When a physician requires a blood test for diagnosis and the client comes to the laboratory with a rolled-up sleeve, consent is being given.

3. A client is scheduled for an office surgical procedure and signs an appropriate consent form. This action constitutes a medical contract between the client and the physician. Written consent has been obtained.

4. If a client who comes to the office suddenly stops breathing during the physician's examination, the physician will take immediate action to restore breathing and prevent any further damage. Consent is

implied by law in an emergency situation when a client is unable to give consent. An emergency is said to exist when the client is in immediate danger and action is necessary to save a life or prevent further damage.

Integral to consent is the client's belief that the health care professional to whom consent is given has the knowledge, skill, and ability to perform such tasks. In our examples, the client has a right to expect that the physician has the ability to determine the need for a throat culture, perform the required surgery, and administer emergency treatment. Likewise, the client can expect the laboratory technician to know proper venipuncture technique.

INFORMED AND UNINFORMED CONSENT

Two underlying reasons for obtaining informed consent are to ensure individual autonomy (the right to be left alone or the right to privacy) and to encourage rational decision making. Consent is a process, not a mere piece of paper or form to sign. The process implies a two-way communication between client and health care provider that will maximize the client's participation.

Ideally, all consent is informed, with the client understanding all facets of the consent. Clients who are a party to consent usually are informed or have sufficient understanding of the circumstances surrounding their consent. **Uninformed consent** occurs when the client gives permission but does not understand or comprehend what has been consented to.

Because of the many occasions arising in the ambulatory health care setting that involve complicated medical procedures that are often difficult for clients to understand, informed consent is important to give the physician permission to act. To ensure that proper consent is obtained, it usually is put in writing. States have specific guidelines generally established in the doctrine of informed consent.

THE DOCTRINE OF INFORMED CONSENT

Informed consent is a client's right to know and understand before agreeing to a procedure. Consent should be obtained in writing because written consent implies an intentional and deliberate decision.

States vary in their informed consent laws but require that the client understand the nature of the illness and be told, in language easily understood, the following:

1. What the procedure is and how it is to be performed
2. The possible risks involved and the expected results
3. Any alternative procedures or treatments and their risks
4. Results if no treatment is given

> To further illustrate the necessary elements of informed consent, consider Phil, age 65, who has been diagnosed by the physician as having adenocarcinoma. His physician is careful to explain the nature of this particular disease to Phil and its possible progression in his body. The physician then outlines the possible forms of treatment, such as surgery, chemotherapy, or radiation, and carefully explains the risks of each, as well as possible outcomes. The physician frequently encourages a particular form of treatment even before the client asks for a recommendation. Here the physician has knowledge of Phil's particular case that may be expected to give credence to such a recommendation. However, the physician should be careful also to explain the possible risks of no treatment at all. Although the client looks to the physician for medical information and recommendations, the decision is the client's alone.

In Phil's situation (see box), as with most others, all office staff members must be sensitive to the impact of such a decision. For consent to be meaningful, Phil may need time to comprehend the essential elements of the consent. This may include talking with family members, seeking a second opinion, considering financial implications, or just being alone. Staff members also need to be prepared to clarify, further explain, or direct additional questions to the physician if the client so indicates. Not until a later time will written consent be obtained and the physician be able to proceed. The written consent must reflect each of the elements described and should also contain the client's signature, the physician's signature, and the signature of a witness.

▆▆▆ PROBLEMS IN CONSENT

Consent may be difficult to obtain in the treatment of a **minor,** a person who has not reached the age of maturity. In some states, courts recognize two types of minors who are capable of informed consent. Mature minors are "judicially recognized as possessing sufficient understanding and appreciation of the nature and consequences of treatment despite their chronological age."[1] Emancipated minors have the legal capacity of an adult when (1) they are living on their own, (2) they are self-supporting, (3) they are married, (4) they are in the armed forces, or (5) any combination of these factors.[2] Legal questions of capacity to consent related to both the **mature minor** and the **emancipated minor** are considered on a case-by-case basis because not all states recognize mature or emancipated minors.

In most states, minors are unable to give consent for medical care except as described previously or in special cases when minors are pregnant, request birth control or abortion, have suspected sexually transmitted diseases, have possible problems with substance abuse, or are in need of psychiatric care. In all other situations, the physician or staff should attempt to reach the parent(s) or legal guardian(s) for consent.

Legal implications to consider when treating a minor are as follows:

1. A minor has the right to confidentiality. A 16-year-old who seeks a prescription for birth control pills has the right for that information to be kept confidential.
2. A minor who may legally consent to treatment may not be financially responsible. If the 16-year-old in the first example does not pay when services are given, collecting from parents who have not given their consent may be difficult and breaches confidentiality.
3. A minor's legal guardian may have to be determined—a special problem in the case of divorce and remarriage. If the father of a child is financially responsible, but the child resides with the mother, who may properly give consent for treatment?

You must be knowledgeable regarding your own state consent laws and have an attorney's recommendations when problems occur.

The law that governs consent is not well defined for minors, and it may be vague or even nonexistent with respect to spouses. Increased awareness of the rights of women has made significant impact on the legal system. More advancements can be expected in the future.

Generally, a spouse has the legal right to consent to and receive medical care and treatment without a spouse's approval. In some situations, however, medical providers may seek consent from both spouses as an additional precautionary measure. Such situations include convenience sterilization and abortion.

CRITICAL THINKING EXERCISE

A 17-year-old ward of the court is pregnant and gives birth to a son. She identifies the father on the birth certificate. Social services garnishes his wages for child support.

Should the father of an unborn child have any say if the mother seeks an abortion instead of giving birth?

Other problems in consent may arise in the case of foster children, stroke clients who cannot communicate, the mentally incompetent (including those in shock and trauma), senile clients, and those temporarily or permanently under the influence of drugs or alcohol. A legal guardian who can give consent may have to be appointed by the courts. The ambulatory health care staff must determine who legally is responsible in each case. When there is immediate danger to life and limb, however, the law implies consent for treatment for these individuals without consent from the responsible party.

Language can be a barrier to informed consent with the increased immigration in this country. An interpreter may be necessary so that information for consent can be given in the native tongue to ensure comprehension.

A number of exceptions to informed consent are peculiar to each state. Examples include the following:

1. The physician may not need to disclose risks commonly known.
2. The physician may not be responsible for failing to disclose risks when the knowledge might be detrimental to the client's best interest.
3. A physician may not need to disclose risks if the client requests to remain ignorant.

A client has the right to refuse treatment. Such is often the case for Christian Scientists or Jehovah's Witnesses, who may refuse medical care or blood transfusions on religious grounds. In some situations, the court appoints a guardian, who then may give consent for the client. This is especially true in the case of minors.

Check your state's doctrine of informed consent for specific exceptions and information. Local medical societies also may offer information.

Vignette 8

Dr. Enke's laboratory technician explains any necessary tests to her clients as a standard procedure. The client, Smoger, was unhappy and thought he would have had much less trouble with his laboratory test had the doctor herself made the explanation.

Outcome: A federal court ruled that a doctor can have a laboratory technician tell a patient about the risks involved in a test, stating, "It violates no requirement of the law for the doctor to delegate the duty to inform."

Note: This vignette is based, in part, on *Smoger v Enke*, 874 F2d 295 (5th Cir 1989).

◼ IMPLEMENTING CONSENT

Consent forms are prepared for the client's signature. The office staff may be responsible for the preparation of specifically designed forms or the procurement of preprinted consent forms (Fig. 7–1). In either case, the form must be understandable, protect the rights of the client, and be broad enough to cover anything contemplated, but specific enough to create informed consent. A so-called blanket consent form, which seeks to cover all aspects of client care and is not specific, must be avoided.

Care should be given to be certain that all elements of informed consent have been understood by the client before a signature is affixed. The consent form should include an expiration date. In some states, 90 days is the maximum. Another consideration may be allowing a waiting period between consent and administration of the procedure or treatment, the latter particularly in the case of sterilization.

The consent process ought to be concisely documented in the medical record. Some physicians tape-record the informed consent process and save the tapes. Others have a checklist for the informed consent interview. Whatever procedures are followed, informed consent should be sought as soon as possible after the need is identified.

An ambulatory health care employee may be asked to witness a signature in order to verify that the signature is indeed that of the client. The physician is responsible for the explanation of medical treatment to the client, even though the employee may provide reinforcement through clarification. If the client has any further questions about the treatment or difficulties with the consent form, let the physician know. If the client signs with an X, two witnesses are required. The younger staff members should

A   **Permission For Diagnostic Procedure:
Verification of Informed Consent**

I hereby authorize and direct_____, M.D., with associates or assistants of his/her choice, to perform the following operation on _____,
my _____ as we have agreed upon: _____Patient_____
　　　　　Self/Relationship
_____

    I further authorize the doctor(s) to do any other procedure that their judgment may dictate to
be necessary or advisable should unforeseen circumstances arise during the procedure. The
details of the procedure have been explained to me in terms that I could understand. Alternative
methods of diagnosis, if any, have been explained to me, as have been the benefits and
disadvantages of each. I also understand the risks, if any, of refusing the procedure. I am advised
that though no complications are expected, they cannot be anticipated and that therefore there
can be no guarantee, either expressed or implied, as to the results of the procedure. The doctor
has answered all my questions.
    The doctor has explained to me the most *likely* complications or problems that might occur
during this procedure and during the healing period, if any, and *I understand them.*
    The doctor has offered to detail the less likely complications which, even if rare, could occur.

Please check one:
_____ *I do wish to have these described to me*　　_____ *I do not wish to have these described to me*

    I understand there is a remote risk of death or serious disability with any procedure.
    I authorize and direct the above-named doctor, with his/her associates or assistants, to provide
such additional services as they may deem reasonable and necessary including, but not limited to,
the administration of any anesthetic agent and the services of the x-ray department and the labo-
ratories.
    I further consent to the administration of such anesthetics as may be considered necessary. I
recognize that there are always risks to life and health associated with anesthesia and such risks
have been fully explained to me.

Please check:
_____ *I certify that I have read and that I understand this consent and that all blanks were filled in prior
to my signature.*

_____　　　_____
　Patient or Legal Guardian Signature　　　　　　　　　　Date

_____　　　_____
　Witnesss　　　　　　　　　　　　　　　　　　　Relationship

I hereby certify that I have explained the nature, purpose, benefits, risks of, and alternatives
to, the proposed procedure, have offered to answer any questions and have fully answered all
such questions. I believe that the patient/relative/guardian fully understands what I have
explained and answered.

_____　　　_____
　Physician Signature　　　　　　　　　　　　　　Date

Note: This document must be made part of the patient's medical records.

Figure 7–1. Informed consent forms: A, for a diagnostic procedure.

B   **Permission For Surgical Care:
Verification of Informed Consent**

I hereby authorize and direct _____, M.D., with associates or
assistants of his/her choice, to perform the following operation on_____,
my _____ as we have agreed upon: _____
Self/Relationship   Patient

I further authorize the doctor(s) to do any other procedure that their judgment may dictate to
be necessary or advisable should unforeseen circumstances arise during the operation. The details
of the operation or procedure have been explained to me in terms that I could understand. Alternative methods of treatment, if any, have been explained to me, as have been the benefits and disadvantages of each. We have also discussed the risks, if any, of not having the operation or procedure. I am advised that though good results are expected, complications cannot be anticipated
and that therefore there can be no guarantee, either expressed or implied, as to the results of the
surgery or cure. The doctor has answered all my questions.

The doctor has explained to me the most *likely* complications or problems that might occur in
this operation and during the healing period, *and I understand them.*

The doctor has offered to detail the less likely complications which, even if rare, could occur.

Please check one:
_____ *I do wish to have these described to me*   _____ *I do not wish to have these described to me*

I understand there is a remote risk of death or serious disability with any procedure.

I authorize and direct the above-named doctor, with his/her associates or assistants, to provide
such additional services as they may deem reasonable and necessary including, but not limited to,
the administration of any anesthetic agent and the services of the x-ray department and the labora-
tories.

I further consent to the administration of such anesthetics as may be considered necessary. I
recognize that there are always risks to life and health associated with anesthesia and such risks
have been fully explained to me.

Please check:
_____ *I certify that I have read and that I understand this consent and that all blanks were filled in prior to
my signature.*

_____	_____
Patient or Legal Guardian Signature	Date
_____	_____
Witnesss	Relationship

I hereby certify that I have explained the nature, purpose, benefits, risks of, and
alternatives to, the proposed procedure/operation, have offered to answer any questions and
have fully answered all such questions. I believe that the patient/relative/guardian fully
understands what I have explained and answered.

_____	_____
Physician Signature	Date

Note: This document must be made part of the patient's medical records.

Figure 7–1. *B*, for a surgical procedure.

C   Refusal to Consent to Treatment

I have been advised by Dr. _____ that the following treatment _____ should be given to me/the below-named patient (please type or print): _____

Dr. _____ has fully explained to me the nature and purposes of the proposed treatment, the possible alternatives thereto and the risks and consequences of not proceeding.

I nonetheless refuse to consent to the proposed treatment.

I have been given an opportunity to ask questions, and all my questions have been answered to my satisfaction.

I hereby release _____ Hospital and its employees, students and medical staff from any liability for any ill effects that I may suffer from failure to perform the proposed treatment.

I confirm that I have read and fully understand the above and that all the blank spaces have been completed prior to my signing.

_____   _____
Patient or Legal Guardian Signature   Date

_____   _____
Witnesss   Relationship

I hereby certify that I have explained the nature, purpose, benefits, and alternatives to, the proposed treatment and the risks and consequences of not proceeding, have offered to answer any questions and have fully answered all such questions. I believe that the patient/relative/guardian fully understands what I have explained and answered.

_____   _____
Physician Signature   Date

Note: This document must be made part of the patient's medical records.

Figure 7–1. C, for refusal to consent to treatment.

witness consent forms; this helps ensure the longevity of the witnesses, should there be any problems in later years. At least three copies of the signed consent form are necessary—one for the client, one for the records, and one for the hospital, if necessary.

REFERENCES

1. Rozovsky, FA: Consent to Treatment: A Practical Guide, ed 2. Little, Brown, Boston, 1990, p 260.
2. Ibid, p 266.

BIBLIOGRAPHY

Dubler, NV, and Minnons, D: Ethics on Call. Harmony Books, New York, 1992.
Farrow, BR, et al: Health Law, Vol. 1. West, St Paul, Minn, 1995.
Health Care Law and Ethics. American Association of Medical Assistants, Chicago, 1996.

Discussion Questions

1. *Define consent and doctrine of informed consent.*
2. *Differentiate between informed and uninformed consent.*
3. *In emergency situations, what type of consent exists? Explain and give an example.*
4. *The parents of a 6-year-old child consented to allow her to undergo "routine cardiac tests." One of the tests performed was a catheter arteriogram in which complications occurred. Questioning the parents revealed that they did not fully understand the risks involved. What are the legal implications of this consent? Identify potential problems in this situation.*
5. *What is the age of maturity in your state?*
6. *A 15-year-old enters your office requesting treatment for scalds received on his hand while emptying the dishwasher at his place of employment. Although his family receives medical treatment at your office, you are uncertain about seeing him without his parents' knowledge. Can he consent to treatment? What are the legal ramifications?*
7. *How specific should a consent form be? How general? Explain.*
8. *When you are asked to witness a signature, what does it legally mean?*

9. *An unmarried pregnant client requests an abortion. Assuming the abortion is legal, what rights, if any, does the father have in consent?*

10. *After a client signed a consent form and you have witnessed it, she states, "I hope this is the right decision." What would you reply? What would you do?*

11. *In your state, is it the responsibility of physicians to obtain the signature for informed consent from clients? Explain. May other health care employees legally obtain the signature for informed consent? Explain.*

chapter 8

Medical Records

LEARNING OBJECTIVES

Upon successful completion of this chapter, you will be able to:

1. Define the term *medical records*.
2. List six purposes of medical records in the ambulatory health care setting.
3. Name and define two types of charting.
4. Define the term *SOAP* and its use in medical records.
5. Demonstrate by example how and when to correct an error in medical records.
6. Define the terms *confidentiality* and *right to privacy* as they relate to medical records.
7. Identify two circumstances in which a release of information is unnecessary.
8. Outline the process to follow when a subpoena is served.
9. Tell who owns medical records.
10. List and define two storage methods for medical records.

DEFINITIONS

Microform. Method of filing data on film using minute images.
POMR. Problem-oriented medical record. A charting system, developed by Lawrence L. Weed, MD, that is based on client problems.
SOAP. A charting method using subjective and objective data for client assessment and planning.

The development and care of medical records require much attention from the ambulatory health care staff. Both employees and physicians collect and enter data into clients' medical records. Medical records are a part of every person's life, beginning with the birth certificate and ending with the death certificate. With increased health awareness, clients are more concerned about what goes into their medical records. Clients also care who has access to their records. Are the records legal documents? Are they confidential? What authorization is required to release clients' medical records? Who owns them? These are questions ambulatory health care employees face daily.

The primary goal of any medical record is the proper care and identification of the client. A client's medical record that is accurate, complete, and concise encourages better medical care than a record that is not up-to-date and is a folder of loose papers not necessarily related or in order.

This chapter deals with medical records in the ambulatory care setting rather than hospital medical records. Although regulations for hospital records may be mandated by state statutes and requirements for hospital licensure, generally regulations for medical records in the ambulatory health care setting are not tied to licensure.

PURPOSES

The Joint Commission on Accreditation of Hospitals has established guidelines for medical records in the hospital.

> Using these as a base, the primary purposes of medical records in ambulatory health care are to
> 1. Provide a base for managing client care, which includes initiating, diagnosing, implementing, and evaluating.
> 2. Provide interoffice and intraoffice communication of client-related data.
> 3. Document total and complete health care from birth to death.
> 4. Allow patterns to surface that will alert physicians of clients' needs.
> 5. Serve as a legal basis for evidence in litigation and to protect the legal interests of clients.
> 6. Provide clinical data for education and research.

The medical record is an official documentation of what has happened to the client during a specific time. The type of charting and medical record used in ambulatory health care settings varies. Specialists who see the client only once may have an abbreviated form of medical record, merely a 5 × 8 inch card. By contrast, a physician who has had the same client for 30 years may have the equivalent of three file folders with several hundred sheets of medical data on that client. Increasingly, medical charts are computerized. Whatever type is used, each client needs a medical record.

PROBLEM-ORIENTED MEDICAL RECORDS

The problem-oriented medical record (**POMR**), or problem-oriented record (**POR**), was developed by Dr. Lawrence L. Weed. The POMR is based on the client's problems, and every ambulatory health care employee, including the physician, charts in a particular place in the same manner. The POMR identifies the client's problems, not simply diagnoses, based on defined data. A problem can be a condition or a behavior that results in physical or emotional distress or interferes with the client's functioning. Examples include pain in the knees and ankles, fear of falling, decreased appetite, and even an inability to pay medical bills. The problem list is usually numbered, appears on the chart face sheet, and serves as a checklist to ascertain the client's progress.

To identify clients' problems, the physician selects a database that may include a physical examination, history, laboratory tests, and subjective data from the client. Every problem has a plan, and its progress is recorded in the medical record.

Weed also developed a computerized medical record that permits the health care provider to build a computer-based POMR while accessing data pertinent to the problem from current literature.

SOAP

Many ambulatory health care settings use **SOAP**—subjective, objective, assessment, and plan—as a method of charting. Once a problem is identified, it is SOAPed.

Subjective includes what the subject or client says, family comments, and hearsay; the client's exact words are recorded.

Objective includes events that are directly observed or measurable, including laboratory tests, roentgenogram results, and physical examination findings.

Assessment includes the physician's evaluation based on the subjective and objective data (S + O = A).

Plan includes the treatment plan and the actions taken.

An example of the SOAP format is shown in Figure 8–1. SOAP also may be found in a source-oriented medical record, which is more likely a collection of narrative pages. Each time the client is seen by the physician, an entry is handwritten by the physician or dictated and then transcribed by an employee. Laboratory and roentgenogram results are collected

CALCANEO, Henry R.
08/18/40

Date of Onset	Date Recorded	PROBLEM LIST	Date Resolved	INACTIVE PROBLEMS
?	10/08/97	1. Increased appetite, increased thirst	10/20/97	
05/28/98	06/30/98		07/10/98	
08/11/98	08/21/98	2. Dyspnea 3. Loss of job		

10/08/97   1. <u>Increased appetite, increased thirst</u>

S: I eat all the time and never gain weight." "I didn't think about it, but yes, I drink all the time, too."

O: B/P 120/88. T--P--R: 98⁹--80--18. Color good. Skin turgor adequate. Wt. 5# less than 3 weeks ago. Urine, 4+ sugar. FBS, positive.

A: Uncontrolled diabetes; in family history.

P: Dx: Lab work-up for diabetes.
Tx: Begin on insulin; Diabetic diet.
Ed: Enroll in diabetic classes stat; instruct in diet and exercise.

06/30/98   2. <u>Dyspnea</u>

S: "I can't seem to get my breath. I'm weak all the time. It's worse when I lay down."

O: B/P 180/98. T--P--R: 99--88--26. Chest x-ray negative. Awakens from sleep with respiratory distress. Cough; slight edema.

A: Congestive heart failure, left sided. History of hypertension and diabetes.

P: Hospitalize for cardiac work-up.

08/21/98   3. <u>Loss of Job</u>

S: "What can I do now? I'm not trained for anything but construction, and with this heart problem, I'll never get back my old job."

O: Heart condition improved; wt. gain 30#; brittle diabetic.

A: Doesn't seem worried about a job; is upset that current job is not available to him now. Off diet.

P: Send to rehab for evaluation and training for new profession; stress diet and exercise; lose 20 lbs.

Figure 8–1. Example of the use of SOAP charting.

together, may be color coded, and may be shingled or layered chronologically.

Whatever method of charting is used in medical records, it must be concise, complete, clear, and in chronologic order.

◼️ USE OF RECORDS IN LITIGATION

Medical records are legal documents and as such become a vital piece of evidence in any malpractice case.

> One method to ensure that medical records present the best documentation of client care is RALTIC.[1] The records should be
>
> Relevant
> Accurate
> Legible
> Timely
> Informative
> Complete

Each state has specific laws regulating the use of medical records. For example, in Washington health care providers and health care facilities are required to provide a notice of information regarding the use of medical records to clients either by posting a sign or sending the notice to clients. The law further specifies what the notice must state:

We keep a record of the health care services we provide you. You may ask us to see and copy that record. You may also ask us to correct that record. We will not disclose your record to others unless you direct us to do so or unless the law authorizes or compels us to do so. You may see your record or get more information about it at _____ Revised Code of Washington, a state statute, RCW 42.17.

Also, more states are enacting legislation regulating disclosure of information about human immunodeficiency virus (HIV) and acquired immunodeficiency syndrome (AIDS). For example, in Washington a separate consent form must be obtained from the client for disclosure of HIV or AIDS information, and a court order is required to authorize disclosure of HIV information. A subpoena is not sufficient. Some states require that information related to HIV and AIDS be maintained in a special manner. Ambulatory health care personnel should establish a protocol for ensuring that the HIV and AIDS information in the medical record complies with applicable state laws.

Physicians and employees should remember that the medical record may be as valuable for what it does not say as for what it does say. An act not recorded is generally considered an act not performed by most courts of law. The necessity for using a medical record in a court emphasizes the importance of accurate records that honestly reflect the client's course of treatment. A record that is readable, understandable, and complete will better withstand scrutiny in a courtroom.

If an error is made on a medical record, it must be properly corrected. Errors made while keyboarding should be corrected as any other keyboarded material would be. Handwritten errors and keyboarded errors discovered later should be corrected by the following method: draw a line through the error, write "correction" or "corr.," sign your initials, indicate the date, and write in the correction. When erasures or obliterations occur, confusion and suspicion may result. Poor or altered records can be detrimental to the physician's defense in court.

The medical record often becomes the center of a malpractice action wherein both attorneys involved will bring in forensic document examiners to investigate the reliability of the record. Such experts will use specialized equipment that can detect different inks in the same entry, which a jury can easily interpret. Scientific equipment also can detect when pages have been added after the fact. Ambulatory health care personnel should never change a medical record unless correcting it properly. Never "leave room" for someone else to chart later. Such a space may cause suspicion rather than a late entry. And never remove a report or note from a medical record because it, too, may indicate that a record has been tampered with.

The medical record is confidential. Any employee handling records must protect the privacy of clients unless otherwise required by law. Some states consider communication between client and physician to be privileged. The privilege belongs to clients and is important because physicians need to know highly personal and private information about clients during the course of treatment.

No information should be released from the medical record without the physician's approval and the written permission of the client, and then only the specific information authorized should be released (Fig. 8–2). Creating a form that may be signed by clients for the release of any medical records may be helpful. The simplest release is seen on many insurance claim forms, which require the client's signature before certain data are released to the insurance carrier.

If the client is a minor, the parent or legal guardian may sign. If the parents are legally separated or divorced, the parent who has legal custody of the minor must sign all release forms. If the client is incompetent, the court-appointed guardian signs the release of information. If the client is deceased, the legal representative of the estate signs. Recent laws have allowed some government and state agencies, such as those that administer the medicaid program, access to medical records without clients' consent. A standard procedure is essential for maintaining confidentiality and good client relations.

There are times during the course of medical practice when a client's chart will be subpoenaed by a court of law. Notify the client when releasing the record in accordance with the subpoena. In some states, the attorney who subpoenas the medical record must notify in writing both the provider and the client and allow 14 days for a response. Unless the origi-

AUTHORIZATION TO RELEASE INFORMATION

Please Print Clearly

Name _____
      (Last)   (First)   (M.I.)

Address _____
      (Street)   (City)   (State)

Phone (_____) _____ Date of Birth _____ Medical Record #_____
I authorize_____ to release medical information from my medical record to
Name of Doctor, Hospital, etc. _____
Address _____
City/State/Zip Code_____

for the purpose of review/examination. I further authorize you to provide such copies thereof as may be requested.
The foregoing is subject to such limitation as indicated below:
☐ Entire record
☐ Specific information:_____
☐ Old records from previous physicians: _____

I give special permission to release any information regarding: (initial on applicable line(s) below)

_____ Substance Abuse _____ Psychiatric/Mental Health Information _____ HIV Information

Reason for request_____
This authorization will automatically expire one year from the date signed. I understand that I may revoke this
content at any time except to the extent that action has been taken in reliance thereon.

Signed _____ Date_____

Witness _____ Date_____

FOR OFFICE USE ONLY

Received_____ Completed By_____
Completed _____ Fee Paid_____
Amount Billed $_____ Amount Due _____

Disclosure Consisted Of _____
_____
_____
_____
_____

Name

Figure 8–2. Sample of a form authorizing the release of information.

nal is subpoenaed, a certified photocopy should be made for the courts. If
the original is subpoenaed, a copy should be made to remain in the office.
An original medical record should be hand delivered to the court clerk and
a receipt obtained. The cost of making copies is usually paid by the person
or agency issuing the subpoena.

It should also be noted that a subpoena may not be sufficient to obtain certain types of medical records. As mentioned earlier, the release of

Date: _____
RE: _____
History #/Date of Birth _____

This is a multiple action form letter with only those items indicated by an "X" being applicable.

IN ANSWER TO YOUR REQUEST FOR MEDICAL INFORMATION

Please see attached medical record copies. NOTE: Request for copies of the entire record will include only the last 2 years of lab work. The attached medical information is CONFIDENTIAL. Subsequent disclosure is not authorized without the specific consent of the patient.

REQUEST FOR ADDITIONAL INFORMATION

☐ Your request is being returned for the following reason(s):
    ☐   We are unable to locate a record of treatment for this individual. Please provide additional information, such as full name of patient at time of treatment, date of birth, history #, or verification of spelling of name. RETURN YOUR REQUEST WITH THE INFORMATION.
    ☐   No record on file for specified dates.
    ☐   Medical information is confidential and can be released only on written consent of patient /patient's legally authorized representative. HAVE THE PATIENT COMPLETE THE ENCLOSED CONSENT AND RETURN YOUR REQUEST WITH THE CONSENT.
    ☐   Authorization date is over 6 months. RETURN YOUR REQUEST WITH A MORE RECENTLY DATED AUTHORIZATION SIGNED BY THE PATIENT/PATIENT'S LEGALLY AUTHORIZED REPRESENTATIVE.
    ☐   The authorization received contained insufficient information for release of the information requested.

☐ Our charge for releasing records directly to the patient/patient's representative is $_____ . If you provide us with the name and address of your new physician, we will send the copies there instead, thereby eliminating the charge. Otherwise, make check payable to_____put patient's name on the check, and return a copy of this letter with check.

☐ Please remit _____, which is our fee for processing your request and photocopying the requested record. Make check payable to_____. reference the patient's name on the check, and return a copy of this letter with check.

☐ Other: _____
_____
_____
_____
_____
_____

Figure 8–2. *(continued)*

information related to HIV and AIDS is an example of a restriction. Drug and alcohol records, sexually transmitted disease records, mental health records, and sexual assault records may be restricted also. Client consent or court order may be required for such release.

CRITICAL THINKING EXERCISES

The medical assistant is catching up on the completeness of the practice's medical records. She notices that the physician wants a transcript of two telephone calls that were not previously recorded. She chooses to record them, dates them when the calls were made, and signs the entry.

A well-informed client discusses with the physician marital problems she is having and says, "Please do not record this in my record."

■ COMPUTERIZED MEDICAL RECORDS

With the increased use of computers in ambulatory health care and in some instances the use of computers for clients' charts, confidentiality and accessibility are issues to be addressed. Computer data are easily accessed and changed. Not all ambulatory health care clinics are computerized; however, with the advent of managed care, computers are helping address the increasing need for client information. Computerized records allow health care professionals to remind clients of appointments and in many cases to track client progress faster and more easily. Less storage space is necessary for computerized files, and files can be more easily retrieved. In some cases, the computerized charts are less likely to be misplaced. Of course, files can be easily deleted from the computer, and some ambulatory health care personnel may be reluctant to make the transition to computerized records. Therefore written procedures ought to be established for adding to or changing data on the computer, including who is authorized to make changes, the time in which changes can take place, and who will be informed of those changes. Procedures should also be developed for purging aged data.

Issues of privacy and confidentiality must be addressed with the increased computerization of medical records. It is more difficult to control the redisclosure of information to others and the abuse that might occur in the uncontrolled use of that information when records are computerized. Variance in state laws may pose problems. When medical information crosses state lines, it is not subject to the same constraints held by the originating state. The medical record itself may be compromised if clients become unwilling to provide complete and accurate information about sensitive issues clients believe may not be held in confidence.

■ FAX MACHINES

The facsimile (fax) machine can be especially useful if health care information is needed more quickly than can be accomplished by mail or phone. Also, more detail can be given by FAX than by phone. There are problems, however. The fax may inadvertently be sent to the wrong destination or retrieved by an unauthorized recipient. Therefore careful attention to confidentiality must be considered when using a fax transmission for client medical records. Office policies should be initiated detailing proper procedures. Consider the following guidelines as suggested by the American Health Information Managers Association (AHIMA):

1. Use the fax machine only when mailed copies or original medical records will not suffice.

2. Use the fax machine only for data necessary for client care encounter, not for routine release of data. Do not fax information to attorney offices, insurance carriers, clients, or other non–health care entities.
3. Use the fax machine only when machines are located in restricted access and secure areas.
4. Obtain appropriate client authorization where required before the release of information.
5. Verify the recipient of the fax, the fax number, and the location of the fax machine. Include a statement to those who might receive the fax in error.
6. Document the reason for any fax transmission and any misdirected fax.

The confidentiality notice to accompany any fax is as follows:

The documents accompanying this telecopy transmission contain confidential information belonging to the sender that is legally privileged. This information is intended only for the use of the individual or entity named above. The authorized recipient of this information is prohibited from disclosing this information to any other party and is required to destroy the information after its stated need has been fulfilled. If you are not the intended recipient, you are hereby notified that any disclosure, copying, distribution or action taken in reliance on the contents of these documents is strictly prohibited. If you have received this telecopy in error, please notify the sender immediately to arrange for return of these documents.[2]

OWNERSHIP OF MEDICAL RECORDS

The accepted rule is that medical records are the property of the person or persons entering the data in them. Physicians are considered the owners of the medical records they have written.

In recent years, clients increasingly have been allowed access to their medical records. Some state medical societies encourage the release of a copy of the medical record to a client. Clients may be expected to make an appointment to obtain that copy and pay reproduction fees. When clients have been denied access to their records, attorneys have been employed to obtain copies of the records. Access should be withheld only when the law prohibits such access, or when, in the physician's opinion, great harm would be done to the client.

Clients who request that their medical records be transferred to another physician should do so in writing. The original record may be retained in the office and the request honored with a photocopy of the complete record or the physician's summary. The continuance of medical records is important in a society that is so mobile. This continuity can be accomplished only with cooperation from physicians. A small fee may be charged for copying the record. The important factor is to release the record promptly so that the client can receive proper care from the new physician.

Again, ambulatory health care employees must be especially cautious with automated medical records. The increased use of computers and word processing equipment in ambulatory health care settings for both financial and health records makes confidential information more accessible. The storage of health data and information has valuable possibilities for improving health care but also may lead to an unnecessary and illegal invasion of clients' privacy.

▰ RETENTION OF MEDICAL RECORDS

How long to retain medical records is not easily established. One guideline indicates that records should be retained until the statute of limitations for acts of medical malpractice has expired so that records are available for any possible litigation. This guideline may require a pediatrician to keep the record for as long as 7 to 10 years beyond the age of maturity.

Physicians probably should keep clients' medical records permanently. However, keeping medical records for 7 to 15 years after clients are no longer seeing the physician or 5 years after the date of last service for deceased clients is probably sufficient. In the future, family medical records may be as important as the individual medical record. Perhaps children should have their deceased parents' medical histories added to their own. Recent medical developments show that medications taken by mothers during pregnancy may affect their children in later years. Much client care for illnesses is directly related to genetic makeup. Without family records, full disclosure and study may be impaired.

These suggestions will cause employees and physicians to cringe when thinking of the warehouse they may have to rent to store all the data collected during the course of their clients' treatment.

▰ STORAGE OF MEDICAL RECORDS

Not all medical records need to be kept in the same location. Active records should be in readiness for physicians. Closed or inactive files usually include records of clients who are no longer being seen by the physician who may have moved away or who have died. These files may be kept in a storage area separate from the current and active files. The office may have storage space or may rent storage space in another location.

■ MICROGRAPHICS

If storage space is at a premium, micrographics may provide a solution. Micrographics is a method of filing data on film using minute (micro) images. The types of **microform** most often used in ambulatory health care are microfilm and microfiche.

Microfilm prints the pertinent information from the medical record on film. A 100-ft roll of 16 mm film is stored in a 4 × 4 × 1 inch container. The material contained in such a container is roughly equivalent to one file drawer of medical records. A piece of equipment called a reader is necessary for viewing the information after it has been microfilmed.

Microfiche is a small sheet of microfilm, about 4 × 6 inch, that contains information to be stored. The process is much the same as microfilm except that the material is on sheets rather than film rolls. Microfiche storage requires less space than does microfilm. Again, additional equipment is necessary to view the information.

Before storing data on any microform, a cost comparison should be done, considering the process and equipment to purchase or rent, as well as the space saved. Other considerations are (1) how long the record is to be kept, (2) how frequently retrieval will be necessary, and (3) the importance of any color coding, which is difficult to reproduce on regular microforms.

Much personnel time is required to prepare files for filming. These tasks are difficult to complete in regular working hours when there are many interruptions. Hiring outside assistance for the task or paying ambulatory health care employees for additional hours may be necessary. Professional firms exist that will convert medical records to a microform for storage. They are able to advise and establish a system appropriate for any particular need.

All persons involved in health care need to know how to manage medical records legally, including record creation, storage, retrieval, release, and disposal. Written office procedures for medical records need to be strictly followed. Handling medical records tends to be tedious and time-consuming, but without proper records client care would be extremely difficult. Medical records are a vital part of ambulatory health care, and employees responsible for their care and upkeep should take pride in the knowledge that their work will be displayed in the medical record for many years to come.

REFERENCES

1. Andress, AA: Manual of Medical Office Management. WB Saunders, Philadelphia, 1996.

2. Miller, C: There's an attorney here to see you. Professional Medical Assistant 29(5):14, 1996.

BIBLIOGRAPHY

Confidentiality of Medical Records in Washington, 1994 edition, Medical Educational Services, Inc., Altonna, Wisconsin, 1994. Presented by Jodi Palmer Long, Sallie Theme, Ross D. Jacobson, David L. Glazer, and Frank E. Cuthbertson.

Grady, ML, and Schwartz, H: Literature Review: Automated Data Sources for Ambulatory Care Effectiveness Research. AHCRP Pub. No. 93-0042. US Dept of Health and Human Services, Rockville, Md, 1993.

Hart, LJ: Alterations to medical records can be detected. Professional Medical Assistant 17(6):19, 1994.

Saunders, JM: Patient Confidentiality. Medicode, Inc., Salt Lake City, Utah, 1996.

Discussion Questions

1. *Compare source-oriented medical records and POMRs.*

2. *While you are preparing the client for the physician, the client picks up the medical record and begins to read it. What do you do?*

3. *The following report was phoned in and charted. "Urinalysis 09/16/9– reveals RBC too numerous to count." When the written report is received, you note it as WBC, not RBC. Properly correct.*

4. *You are preparing a medical record after it has been subpoenaed. Describe the procedures you would follow.*

5. *A client becomes angry when refused permission to hand carry medical records when moving out of state. What alternatives can an employee suggest?*

6. *Describe what might be done when there is simply no room for any more medical records in the office.*

7. *Discuss the effects of computerization on medical records.*

9

Collection Practices

LEARNING OBJECTIVES

Upon successful completion of this chapter, you will be able to:

1. Explain, in a short paragraph, the importance of collections.
2. List three guidelines for collections established by the Medical Group Management Association.
3. List at least five appropriate items to be covered in a collection policy.
4. Identify the seven appropriate procedures to follow when collecting a bill by telephone or by mail.
5. Identify the seven "collection dont's" established by the Federal Trade Commission.
6. Explain the one important procedure to follow if a client is denied credit because of a poor credit rating.
7. List nine steps to follow in selecting a collection agency.
8. Write a brief paragraph describing how personal feelings about individuals' ability to pay may influence their care.

The collection of accounts belongs mostly to the business aspect of the ambulatory health care setting. Many physicians believe that discussing financial matters with their clients is not appropriate and prefer not to be involved with the day-to-day task of collections. Medical health care employees generally avoid the task as long as possible, believing that collections do not deserve the same level of importance as does direct client care.

However, clients may become dissatisfied over collection of a fee more readily than over negligence. A reason for this may be that clients often protect their money more than their personal well-being. Many clients have been angered over an incorrect statement, a change to computer billing that prints overdue notices, or a situation in which an ambulatory health care employee cannot answer financial questions over the telephone.

Physicians are expected to treat the person rather than collect the bill, and they may not have time to devote to the financial practices of the office. Yet every health care employee knows how important the total of the month's receipts is to the physician. Medical health care employees who believe this task has less importance than direct client care should remember that financial dealings with the client allow them to care for the "whole" person. Many lawsuits have their inception in the front office over financial matters. Therefore discussing collections is appropriate.

The days of physicians rendering their services in exchange for a dozen eggs or wood for their stoves are gone. Asking for cash payment at the time services are provided is increasingly popular. Additionally, more and more offices accept credit cards as payment, thus avoiding the problem of collections entirely. Physicians have a right to be reimbursed for the services they perform. Many years of training and education have been required to allow them to practice medicine. Their office equipment and supplies are costly. Physicians and their employees should not hesitate to charge adequate fees for services rendered. An honest discussion with clients before providing services is essential. Clients want to know what is expected of them financially. Being able to give clients a written statement regarding payment for services, insurance reimbursement, and collection policies is most helpful.

■■■■ TRUTH IN LENDING ACT

Regulation Z of the Consumer Protection Act of 1968 is also known as the Truth in Lending Act. This act is enforced by the Federal Trade Commission, and when applied to medical offices it deals with collection of clients' payments.

Briefly, the regulation requires that an agreement by physicians and their clients for payment of medical bills in more than four installments must be in writing and must provide information regarding finance charges. Even if no finace charge is involved, the agreement must be in writing and stipulate no finance charge.

If consumers decide to pay their bills by installments unilaterally with no established agreement with physicians, Regulation Z is not applicable so long as the physician's office continues to bill for the full amount.

Situations in which the Truth in Lending Act is often used include arrangements for surgery and prenatal or delivery care. The amount owed by the client is often more than a client can pay in one installment or is more than is covered by medical insurance. Office employees then can discuss with the client appropriate installment payments, put the agreement in writing, and provide a copy for the client. Few physicians will charge a finance fee in this situation, although to do so is both legal and ethical. If bilateral installment agreements are common in your ambulatory health care clinic or if computer billing automatically includes a finance charge after a certain period, have the wording approved by a legal representative.

◼◼ COLLECTION GUIDELINES

The Medical Group Management Association suggests three guidelines for collections that are worth noting:
1. Collections must provide enough money to maintain the clinic and satisfy the physicians.
2. Collection procedures must be firm enough to be effective.
3. Collections must be temperate enough not to irritate otherwise satisfied consumers who intend to pay.

The guidelines do not discuss how to establish fees, but if the physicians' fees are consistent with those charged by others in the same community who perform similar tasks, clients are unlikely to feel that their bills are unreasonable. Physicians should not hesitate to discuss directly with consumers the fees for their services. Many times, a client more readily accepts a statement of fees from a doctor than from an office assistant.

Medical offices must establish an appropriate collection policy for employees to follow. Clients need to be informed in writing of the policy. That policy should state how insurance claims are handled. Will the office file claims for all insurance carriers, or only a certain few? The policy should state how and when co-payments and deductibles are collected. Does your office charge for completing insurance forms? The policy should determine whether and at what point collection letters will be sent. Will they be printed forms or personal letters? Will there be a minimum payment schedule? Will the letter be different for every account? Are collection telephone calls to be made? If so, by whom? How many? When? What procedures will be followed? Will delinquent accounts ever be turned over to a collection agency or pursued through the local courts? A clearly defined or stated policy gives employees the support necessary for successful collections.

◼◼ COLLECTION DO'S

The following guidelines are provided to suggest possible procedures for collections in the ambulatory health care setting:

1. Establish appropriate fees for the services rendered in accordance with community guidelines and practices.

2. Discuss fees with consumers the first time they present themselves at the office or call for treatment. A written payment policy is essential.

3. Expect first-time clients to pay cash at the end of their visit.

4. Provide clients with an office brochure that gives them information about hours, emergency contacts, physicians' services, how billing is handled, and whom to call if there is a question about a bill. The brochure also should describe how insurance is handled.

5. Provide an opportunity for the client to pay before leaving the office. The charge slip is an ideal way for the physician to circle charges and services rendered, as well as the diagnoses. The bill then is presented to clients, who are asked to stop at the receptionist's desk on their way out. The receptionist should never say, "Shall we bill you?" The receptionist should say, "Mrs. Lotta M. Bucks, your charge today is $65.00. Would you like to pay by cash or check?" Some offices have been successful in providing clients with a stamped, addressed envelope in which to mail the fee when they return home. Other offices do their first billing when the client is ready to leave rather than at the end of the month.

6. If your office uses computer billing, explain the process to the clients. Notify them when you move to a computer system so that they will understand the changes and any problems that may occur.

7. Have an established practice for mailing your statements, and follow that practice. Statements should be itemized, accurate, and easy to understand. Make sure all credits have been posted up to closing date. They should be mailed to arrive the first of the month. Statements that include envelopes, especially colored ones, are paid faster.

8. When your collection policy dictates that a bill should be followed with a letter or a telephone call, do it. Be consistent, pleasant, and firm. The sooner you follow up on a delinquent account, the more likely it will be collected.

9. Employees responsible for collections should have certain phrases and the wording of possible letters at their fingertips for quick and easy referral. They also need the authority to carry the collection process to its completion.

10. Suggested procedures for mail or telephone follow-up include the following: (a) Introduction or greeting. (b) Establish that you are speaking to the proper person, if it is a telephone call, or address the letter to the proper person. (c) State the reason for the call or the letter. ("Your account is past due.") (d) Be pleasant, but be firm. ("You are generally prompt with your payments; we wondered if this has been overlooked.") (e) Get a commitment. Make it specific. ("May we expect $35 from you by next Monday?") Then mark that commitment in

your tickler file and follow up next Monday if there has been no response. (f) End the contact graciously. Do not get pulled into all the financial problems of the client. (g) Be prepared to offer a payment plan that is suitable both to the client and to the physician.

11. Have a clearly established practice of when, if ever, to turn the account over to a collection agency, to collect the balance due in small claims court, or to write off the balance as a loss.

▰▰▰ COLLECTION DONT'S

The Federal Trade Commission has specific regulations for debt collection. They include the following:

1. Do not misrepresent who you are or why you are contacting a person.
2. Do not send "blind" postcards or notices saying, "Please call me," signed "Janet."
3. Do not use deception in any form in your contact.
4. Do not telephone at odd hours or make repeated calls or calls to the debtor's friends, relatives, neighbors, employers, or children. Acceptable hours to call are 8 AM to 8 PM.
5. Do not threaten or falsely assert that credit ratings will be hurt.
6. Do not make calls or send letters demanding payment for amounts not owed.
7. If a contact must be made to the debtor's place of business, do not reveal to a third party the reason for the contact. The client's privacy and reputation must be protected.

If your office denies credit to a client on the basis of an adverse credit report from a credit bureau or similar agency, you must volunteer the name and address of the agency providing the information to the client, even if you are not asked. Failure to do so could result in legal action. Let clients know that it is their right to obtain a copy of their credit report to see if all the information is correct. A form letter should be available in your office that courteously informs the client that credit has been denied, leaving blanks for the name and address of the agency that supplied the credit information. Mail a copy to the client and keep a copy for your records.

▰▰▰ COLLECTION PROBLEMS

An up-front, matter-of-fact approach to collections will increase the cash flow in the ambulatory health care setting and make collections easier for everyone. However, every office has slow payers, hardship cases, and deadbeats. Try to move slow payers to a cash basis as soon and as often as possible and yet maintain good public relations.

Hardship cases pose another problem. Any of us could reach a time in our lives when the payment of a medical bill might be nearly impossible. Care must be taken to be understanding at all times. Try to work out minimal payment plans with the clients so that they, too, are able to take pride in themselves and their ability to pay. Social agencies may be suggested if necessary. If circumstances dictate, physicians may choose to write off an account rather than try to collect. That is a decision for the physician.

The deadbeat is still another problem. There will always be a small percentage of clients who never intend to pay their bills. All possible resources should be exhausted in a courteous manner, but the accounts then should be taken to small claims court or turned over to a collection agency. Physicians often withdraw themselves formally from these cases and encourage the clients to seek treatment elsewhere.

Chapter 4 gives information about the procedures to follow for collecting a bill from the estate of a client who has died. Also in Chapter 4 is an explanation of the steps to follow for taking a client to small claims court. Both of these situations are fairly uncomplicated and will produce results worth the effort if employees are consistent and conscientious in these dealings.

CRITICAL THINKING EXERCISES

Your employer approaches you and says you are way behind in paying your medical bills. He asks if that is true. What collection tip has been violated?

You are an insurance biller for a large clinic. You delay calling a large family who are clients of your practice. You know they will involve you in a complex, "hard luck" story that probably is true.

COLLECTION AGENCIES

If you have diligently followed your billing and collection procedures and come to the conclusion that the client is not going to pay, you have two options. One option is to write off the account; the other is to turn it over to a collection agency.

Obviously, this decision must be consistent with office policy while still leaving the final decision to the physician. Collection agencies generally are employed as a last resort. Most people, including clients and physicians, tend to have a negative attitude toward collection agencies. However, the agency can be valuable to physicians who choose to use such professional services.

Selection of an appropriate agency should be made as carefully as one would choose a bank. Questions to ask include the following:

1. Does it handle medical and dental accounts exclusively?
2. What methods does it use to collect?
3. What is the agency's financial responsibility?
4. What percentage will the ambulatory health care setting receive?
5. How promptly does it settle accounts?
6. Does the agency have a good bank reference?
7. How much cost versus goodwill will your office incur by using this agency?
8. Will it provide you with a list of satisfied customers or references?
9. Will you have the ability to end the agency's collection efforts?

Check with the Better Business Bureau or the local medical society for possible recommendations. An agency that is a member of the American Collectors Association will generally adhere to high ethical standards.

Once the agency is selected, all the delinquent accounts need to be turned over to it, including any useful nonclinical data. The medical office should keep a record of what has been given to the agency, as well as a running account of the agency's progress. Any contact, whether in person, via phone, or via letter, should cease once the account has been turned over to the collection agency. If the client sends payment to the office, report it immediately to the agency. If clients call, courteously refer them to the agency.

The collection agency is representing the physician and medical staff. Office employees should work with the agency to collect the accounts. Consistent high rates of success by an agency in collecting accounts may be a sign that the ambulatory health care staff lacks sufficient training to be effective in collections.

■■■ COLLECTIONS AND ATTITUDES

The clients' financial status has no bearing on the kind of treatment they should receive in the ambulatory health care setting. The medicaid client should receive the same care as the client who pays cash. Physicians and employees need to be careful of their attitudes toward those clients who have difficulty paying their bills, for whatever reason. Actions often speak louder than words, and clients easily perceive their true meanings.

BIBLIOGRAPHY

Andress, AA: Saunders Manual of Medical Office Management. WB Saunders, Philadelphia, 1996.

Staads, J: Collection control in three steps. Professional Medical Assistant 26(3):6, 1993.

Discussion Questions

1. *As a newly employed medical office manager, you discover that one of the physicians in the office does not follow the written collections policies and is more lenient about clients paying their bills. What problem does this create for you and the other physicians?*

2. *A physician overhears the receptionist say to a client, "Well, you know, we can take only so many welfare clients." How can the client now be put at ease?*

3. *The office has just converted to computer billing. A client encloses a note with a check that says, "Now I guess I'm just a number in your office, too. I don't like your new bills." What course of action would you suggest?*

4. *Correct the following telephone conversation:*

Bookkeeper (BK):	"Hi, this is Dr. Erythro's office. Who's this?"
Client (CL):	"This is Laura Phagocyte."
BK:	"You owe us forty-six dollars and twenty cents. Can you pay us ten dollars today?"
CL:	"Yeah. I'll put it in the mail."
BK:	"Will it be check or money order?"
CL:	"Check."
BK:	"Fine, I'll expect it in a few days. Thank you. Good-bye."

chapter

10 Employment Practices

LEARNING OBJECTIVES

Upon successful completion of this chapter, you will be able to:

1. Explain, in your own words, the importance of correct hiring practices.
2. Recall one source of information on hiring practices beneficial to physicians.
3. List at least four necessary components of personnel policies.
4. Identify the three necessary elements of job descriptions.
5. Discuss office hours, workweek, benefits, and salaries.
6. Explain, in your own words, where and how to locate prospective employees.
7. List eight techniques for effective interviews.
8. Identify the five potential discrimination problems to consider when hiring.
9. Describe sexual harassment, Occupational Safety and Health Act, and Americans with Disabilities Act as federal mandates.
10. Recall procedures for selecting the right employee.
11. Recognize steps that encourage employee longevity.

Physicians do not function alone in the ambulatory health care setting. Even physicians starting practice hire an assistant as soon as possible. Selecting appropriate personnel is an important business task. Present health care employees commonly are influential or directly involved in the process of hiring additional employees. Hiring and preparing employees to function in specific roles are both expensive and time-consuming tasks. It is important to perform the tasks effectively the first time. Major areas of consideration and tasks to perform include the following:

1. Establish personnel policies.
2. Determine job descriptions for each position.

3. Locate the best employee for the job.
4. Conduct effective interviews.
5. Select candidates to fulfill the office needs.
6. Keep employees for the long term.
7. Evaluate employees on a predetermined and regular basis.

▬▬ PERSONNEL POLICIES

Without established personnel policies, physicians soon lose control of the management of their own practices. Before the first person is hired, physicians must determine their office needs, job descriptions, office hours and workweek, benefits and salaries, and how employees will be evaluated. Physicians will want to determine if their employees are to be generalists or specialists in their skills, or if a combination of employees would be more effective.

Once these personnel policies have been determined, they should be set in writing in a policy manual. The policies should be updated from time to time to reflect any changes in the office, but they should always be in writing and available to employees. Once personnel policies have been established, prospective employees' questions can be answered.

If the office policy manual is not intended to be a contract between the employer and the employee, but simply a guideline, the manual should clearly state that its terms do not constitute a contract.

▬▬ JOB DESCRIPTIONS

Job descriptions indicate minimum qualifications required, a description of the jobs to be performed, and to whom the employee is responsible. Written job descriptions are often shared with candidates at the time of interviews.

Job descriptions are developed for each position when a new job is created. A job description must be written. Other medical offices or office managers may be willing to share job descriptions used in their office. Medical assistant educators and professional organizations can also be helpful resources.

The established ambulatory health care clinic will find its employees to be the best resources when writing job descriptions. Job descriptions are established by having the employees put in writing descriptions of the tasks they perform in a normal workday. This exercise provides the basis for the job descriptions.

Office hours and the workweek are generally easier to establish than job descriptions. Hours may be determined by the medical specialty, as well as the dictates of the community. The long and often inconsistent hours of a medical practice should be addressed; for example, will every employee stay late, will hours be staggered, and will overtime be compensated? Will the workweek be the same as or longer than office hours? How will a policy be established that provides for the needs of clients and allows all tasks to be performed?

Many employees become unhappy when they are told upon hiring that the workweek will be 40 hours and then it turns out to be closer to 50 or 60 hours. Planning for overtime is essential. Being honest with employees is a must. Employees must plan for their out-of-office responsibilities so that they do not interfere with the office practice. Day care issues and family needs require firm policies on overtime.

▓▓ BENEFITS AND SALARIES

Benefits and salaries are of concern to both employees and employers. Physicians will want to pay a salary that is commensurate with the responsibilities of the task to be performed and that reflects the education, training, and experience of the employees. A third consideration can be the prevailing wage of the community.

Benefits to consider include medical, sick leave, vacations, holidays, retirement, and profit-sharing plans. Other incentives may include payment of educational courses and seminars and a uniform allowance. An important benefit, especially in the city, may be free parking or bus passes.

▓▓ THE EMPLOYMENT PROCESS

Locating Employees

A valuable resource for ambulatory health clinics seeking employees is the county medical society. Some medical societies sponsor a medical employment agency. Schools in the community that have accredited training programs for medical assistants and medical secretaries often have names of graduates seeking employment.

Professional organizations such as the American Association of Medical Assistants, a national organization for medical office assistants that may have a local chapter in your community, may be able to provide possible candidates for employment.

Other physicians and their employees often know of potential candidates. Employment agencies specializing in medical and dental employment are other sources. Newspaper advertising may also be successful.

In an established medical practice, the initial screening of candidates is often delegated to an office manager or a specific person other than the physician.

Interview Process

With a printed job description and a list of possible candidates, the interview process can begin. The interview is a time to meet with each candidate personally. A job application may or may not have been completed at this point.

Commonsense techniques to make the interview more effective include the following:

1. Identify the purpose of the interview and follow through with it.
2. Avoid interruptions during the interview. Do not rush.
3. Use effective communication skills and listen carefully to the candidate.
4. Match the candidate to the job. Look at the total qualifications of the candidate. Do not pick a clone. Look for diversity.
5. Observe nonverbal behavior.
6. Ask each candidate the same questions. These may include the following: What are your qualifications? Why are you leaving your present position? When can you begin work? What salary do you expect? What do you expect to be doing in 1 year? In 5 years? Why do you want to work here? Do you foresee any difficulties that may prevent you from doing a good job? What prompted you to become a medical employee? What is your major strength? Your major weakness?
7. Remain objective.
8. Maintain control of the interview.
9. Use possible scenarios requiring a solution to help determine skill level and communication style.
10. End on a positive note, summarize, allow for questions from the candidate, and provide the candidate with a possible date for a decision.

After the interview, take the time to make notes that will serve as a reminder later when considering several candidates.

Selecting Employees

After completion of the interview process, make a careful study of all the candidates and their responses to questions. Employment applications should be read, and references should be contacted. Talking with former employers and individuals named as references is an important part of the decision-making process.

How each candidate will function with other staff members should be considered. If candidates have been asked to perform any skill functions, the tests should be checked for accuracy. Candidates may be asked to do some keyboarding, take a spelling test (medical and nonmedical words), or perform a clinical function. Telephone candidates or ask them to telephone the office at a later time to screen their telephone personalities. The manner in which candidates handle the telephone is important because the client's first contact with the doctor is often over the telephone.

Once a decision is made, all candidates should be informed. This is a courtesy often overlooked. Establish a probationary period for the new employee; 3 months is usually adequate time to determine whether or not the working relationship is a good one. At the end of this period, either employee or employer should be free to end the employment agreement. Salary paid during the probationary period may be less than is offered on permanent employment.

Employee Evaluations

Evaluation of employees is an ongoing task throughout the individual's employment. Probably the biggest mistake made in health care employment is not making evaluation a formal process. A clearly established and written evaluation policy and form should be developed and carefully explained to employees. A copy of the evaluation policy and form should also be available to employees. At regular intervals during the course of employment, managers should conduct evaluations. New employees should be evaluated at 3 months, thus ending the probationary period. Another evaluation is conducted 6 months later. Thereafter, yearly evaluations on the date of original hire are conducted. If problems surface or an employee is assigned a new major responsibility, evaluations may increase in frequency. Strengths and weaknesses should be documented. The evaluation then should become part of the employee's personnel file.

An adequate evaluation enables employees to improve job performances, serves as a tool for employers to discuss salary increases, provides background for any necessary dismissal, and establishes a record for future referral. Note the sample patterned after a progress review from *The Business Side of Medical Practice* (Fig. 10–1). Although the evaluation records may assist a manager in determining salary increases, a change in salary is best handled at the end of each year and discussed with each employee. Salary changes and evaluations should be kept separate. However, a wise manager recognizes the value of an excellent employee and will make the salary reimbursement an encouragement for the employee to remain with the practice.

PROGRESS REVIEW

Name _____

Position _____

Date Hired _____

Starting Salary _____

Job Knowledge	Thoroughly understands all aspects.	More than adequate knowledge of job.	Has sufficient knowledge to do job.	Insufficient knowledge of some phases.	Continually needs instruction/supervision.
Comments:					
Quality of Work	Always neat. Accurate and thorough.	Only a few mistakes—careful worker.	Work is acceptable.	Occasionally careless—needs checking.	Inaccurate and careless.
Comments:					
Cooperation	Exceptional team worker: flexible.	Usually agreeable. Tactful and obliging.	Goes along satisfactorily.	Sometimes difficult to work with.	Works poorly with others.
Comments:					
Responsibility	Accepts all responsibilities fully; meets emergencies.	Conscientiously tries to fulfill job responsibilities.	Accepts but does not seek responsibility.	Does some assigned tasks reluctantly.	Often indifferent; avoids responsibilities.
Comments:					

Figure 10–1. Employee evaluation form. (Adapted from American Medical Association: The Business Side of Medical Practice. Monroe, Wisconsin, 1979, pp 73–74.)

Initiative	Self-starter: makes practical suggestions.	Proceeds on assigned work voluntarily and readily accepts suggestions.	Does regular work without prompting.	Relies on others; needs help getting started.	Must usually be told exactly what to do.
Comments:					
Quantity of Work	Maintains high output.	Usually does more than expected.	Does required work.	Inclined to be slow.	Others may need to help complete work.
Comments:					
Dependability	Places company interests ahead of personal conveniences.	Punctual—does not waste time.	Generally on the job as needed.	Some abuses— occasionally needs to be admonished.	Abuses work schedule often.
Comments:					
Leadership/ Supervision	Exceptional leader and organizer.	Poised and is respected by other workers.	Has adequate leadership qualities.	Shy; needs leadership development.	Not an organizer. Does not inspire others.
Comments:					

Figure 10–1. *(continued)*

In What Ways Has This Individual Definitely Grown? _____

What Are the Strong Points? _____

In What Way Has the Individual Failed to Grow? _____

What Are the Weak Points? _____

Days Absent This Period _____

    Office Time (Paid) _____

    Own Time (Non-Paid) _____

    Number Sick Days _____

This Review for the Period _____ to _____ 19 _____

Complete if Employee Is Leaving The Office: Would You Recommend Rehire   _____ (Yes)

    _____ (No)

Why? _____

Reviewing Physician/Administrator: _____   Discussed with Employee on:

_____ (Date)

Figure 10–1. (continued)

Employee Termination

When evaluating employees, the decision may be made to terminate an employee. Termination is a difficult, unpleasant situation, but steps must be taken to protect the practice and to minimize the stress for the employee who is terminated.

If the evaluation process has been effective, documentation exists in the employee's personnel file detailing the problem behaviors. The file should include dates the problems were discussed with the employee and specific actions discussed for correction of the problems. It is best to have the employee sign the documents to ensure that the employee has been informed and understands the problem areas and what specific actions are required for correction. Such written documentation will be essential should the terminated employee later seek litigation.

The employee's progress or lack of progress should be evident in the personnel file. Termination should take place during the probationary period if possible. Warnings to the employee help ward off surprise when termination is made. During the termination conference, it is best to be brief, to the point, and honest without degrading the employee.

Managers can learn from the termination experience. Was the job description clear and accurate? Was the probationary period long enough? Was the evaluation process fair, clear, and well documented? How and when were the problem areas communicated to the employee? However unfortunate termination is to both the employee and employer, it is best to use good human relation skills, express empathy, and communicate clearly your expectations to employees.

Keeping Employees

Keeping employees is as important as selecting them. Salaries that are commensurate with work performance and the qualifications of employees are a must. Salary is not a place to try to cut office expense. The old adage "You get what you pay for" is true in employment.

As important to employees as an adequate salary is the assurance that their work is appreciated and is necessary for efficient functioning in the ambulatory health care setting. "Thank you" and "Well done" are compliments that foster goodwill and motivate employees to greater effectiveness. Good employees merit your trust and increased responsibilities. Encourage employees to improve their education and knowledge, and provide incentives for that. If employees are to be corrected or disciplined, never do so in front of other employees or clients. Most will accept tactful criticism well. Few will forget if they are embarrassed before their peers or the clients. Remembering birthdays and employment anniversaries with simple gifts or cards takes little effort but does much for employee morale.

Employees in the ambulatory health care setting can make or break a medical practice. Take the time and effort to ensure that the office staff functions as a team to create an atmosphere conducive to good physician-client relationships.

CRITICAL THINKING EXERCISES

The office manager in a busy medical practice faces the following hiring situations:

1. A transcriptionist is wheelchair bound. The physician groans, "Isn't there someone else? Do you realize the accommodations we'll have to make?"
2. A medical assistant who is morbidly obese is interviewed. The receptionist sarcastically comments, "That's a good role model to have in a cardiologist's office."
3. A female comments to the only male employee in the medical practice, "You know, when we first hired you, I was concerned. But you complement our practice more than any other medical assistant we have ever had."

LEGAL IMPLICATIONS

Individuals involved in the hiring process need to be knowledgeable of state and federal work and employment regulations. The Department of Labor, Wage, and Hour Division will answer questions regarding minimum wages, use of child labor, and length in work. Your state human rights commission can answer questions on possible discrimination in the interview or hiring process.

The federal law states that an employer of 15 or more people must not discriminate on any form of application for employment. The discrimination includes age, sex, race, creed, marital status, national origin, color, or handicaps (sensory, mental, or physical). State laws may be more strict than federal law. For example, in the state of Washington an employer of eight or more cannot discriminate.

Nothing in either the federal or state discrimination laws is intended to prevent the employer from hiring only the most qualified person. Obviously, to protect this right, a well-written job description is essential.

Potential discrimination problem areas include the following:

1. Age: any inquiry implies a preference and is prohibited.
2. Marital status: no inquiries permitted.
3. Race or color: no inquiry concerning race or color of skin, hair, eyes, and so forth permitted.

4. Sex: no inquiry permitted.
5. Handicap: no inquiry if handicaps or health problems not related to job performance. If the employer needs to take a handicap into account in determining job placement or fitness to perform, an inquiry can be made.

Most laws permit employers to talk about the job, its duties, and its responsibilities but prohibit any questions unrelated to the job. For example, it is not job related to note that the applicant has children, but it is job related to note whether the applicant indicated problems getting to work or working overtime.

Managers preparing for an interview bring a structured outline of subjects to cover with all applicants. Treat the candidates alike in all respects.

Valid reasons for declining applicants include the following:

1. Applicant has health problem that would preclude the safe and efficient performance of the job.
2. Applicant is not fully available for the work schedule of the particular job (observance of religious holidays not included).
3. Insufficient skills training or experience to perform the duties of the particular job.
4. Another applicant is better qualified.[1]

Even though the ambulatory health care setting may not have 15, or even 8, employees, it is best to follow the state and federal requirements, not only for protection but also for ethical reasons and for good public relations.

Sexual Harassment

Sexual harassment may occur on the job. Title VII of the Civil Rights Act of 1964 protects employees from sexual harassment. The Office of Equal Employment Opportunities guidelines make the employer strictly liable for the acts of supervisory employees, as well as for some acts of harassment by co-workers and clients of the company. Written policy on sexual harassment, detailing inappropriate behavior and stating specific steps to be taken to correct an inappropriate situation, should be established.

The traditional form of harassment is the scenario in which sexual favors are implicit and demanded of an employee of a supervisor in exchange for job advancement. This is known in legal terms as *quid pro quo,* which means "this for that." For example, the physician says to an employee, "You know, there's a hefty raise for you if you spend the weekend on my boat." A second, probably more common, form of harassment occurs when the work environment interferes with the employee's work performance. This may take the form of a series of sexual questions, com-

> The office policy should include at least the following:
> 1. A statement that sexual harassment of employees will not be tolerated.
> 2. A statement that an employee who feels harassed needs to bring the matter to the immediate attention of a person designated in the policy.
> 3. A statement about the confidentiality of the incident and specific disciplinary action against the harasser.
> 4. The procedure to follow when harassment occurs.

ments, jokes, or inappropriate touchings by co-workers. For example, a male physician's assistant is always making comments in the front office about "my girls," teasing them about PMS and telling them of their inferiority. When the harassment is commonplace and the supervisor or employer does not correct the situation, the employer is liable under Title VII.

Generally, the easiest way to end harassment is to tell the harasser to stop the behavior. This works in some cases. Telling another colleague or threatening the harasser that you will tell another person is the second-best tactic. Ignoring the offensive behavior does not work. If the harassment continues, employers must make it easy and safe for the harassed to seek help.

Occupational Safety and Health Act

Congress passed the Occupational Safety and Health Act to prevent workplace disease and injuries. This statute applies to virtually every U.S. employer. The general purpose of the act is to require all employers to ensure employee safety and health.

> The Occupational Exposure to Hazardous Chemicals Standard requires the following:
> 1. Inventory any and all hazardous chemicals regarding quantity, manufacturer's name, address, and chemical hazard classification.
> 2. Assemble material safety data sheets (MSDS) from manufacturers. The sheets are kept in a manual and reviewed regularly. The chemicals are labeled using the National Fire Protection Association's color and number method.
> 3. Provide educational training to all employees who handle any hazardous chemicals within 30 days of employment and before an employee is allowed to handle the chemicals.
> 4. Develop and evaluate a chemical hygiene plan to address how to handle any spills or exposures.

There are two standards in the regulations: the Occupational Exposure to Hazardous Chemicals Standard and the Bloodborne Pathogen Standard.

The Bloodborne Pathogen Standard became effective in 1992. Its goal primarily is to reduce occupational-related cases of HIV and hepatitis B infection among health care workers.

The Bloodborne Pathogen Standard addresses the following:

1. Control of and determination of exposure
2. Universal precautions
3. Hepatitis B virus vaccine
4. Postexposure follow-up
5. Labeling and disposal of biologic wastes
6. Housekeeping and laundry functions
7. Employee training for safety and documentation

For the safety of employees and all clients, carefully following and monitoring these regulations is essential. Job descriptions should identify any position that may cause exposure to hazardous chemicals and bloodborne pathogens.

The Occupational Safety and Health Administration (OSHA) is authorized to do the following:

1. Encourage employers and employees to reduce workplace hazards and to implement new and improved health programs.
2. Establish "separate but dependent responsibilities and rights" for employers and employees for the achievement of better safety and health conditions.
3. Maintain a reporting record-keeping system to monitor job-related injuries and illnesses.
4. Develop mandatory job safety and health standards and enforce them effectively.[2]

OSHA may make unannounced visits to the workplace and may issue citations or penalties of up to $1000 per violation to an employer who does not provide a safe environment.

Americans with Disabilities Act

The Americans with Disabilities Act (ADA) was passed in Congress in 1990 to eliminate discrimination in employment against a qualified individual with a disability. The statute applies to all persons with substantial impairment that significantly limits a major function. This includes hearing, seeing, speaking, walking, breathing, performing manual tasks, caring for oneself, learning, and working. It also protects persons with a history of cancer in remission, persons with a history of mental illness, and persons with AIDS or who are HIV positive.

If an employee who is disabled meets *all* the qualifications of the job, the employee must make "reasonable" accommodation for the disability. The employer is not required to make an accommodation that imposes "undue hardship" or requires an action with significant difficulty or expense.

Accommodations might include the following:

Handicap parking
Ramps or elevators
Electronic or easily opened doors
Hallways with at least 36 inches of clearance
Accessible bathroom and lunchroom facilities
Reception counters low enough for a wheelchair (34 inches maximum)

For example, if the best-qualified applicant for receptionist has permanent and serious facial scarring, the applicant cannot be denied the position simply because of the fear of "negative reactions" from others. A transcriptionist in a wheelchair, the best candidate for the job, should be hired. In all probability, reasonable accommodation can be made for this individual.

The employment provisions of the ADA are enforced under the same policies of discrimination under Title VII. Remedies may include hiring, reinstatement, back pay, and the order to stop discrimination.

Most employers with the foresight to hire persons with disabilities and to make the necessary accommodations have found that those employees are among the best.

▰▰ SUMMARY

Outside of concern for appropriate client care, treatment, and comfort, the most important function of the manager and physician will be hiring employees and keeping them. It has been shown that legal implications are far reaching and essential to the process.

State laws and regulations of employees must be considered. Some states regulate medical assistants or require their certification to practice. Some states require a license, a registration, or a certification for certain special or invasive procedures that medical assistants perform. The certified medical assistant is one who has graduated from a CAAHEP-accredited educational program and has successfully passed the national certification examination prepared by the American Association of Medical Assistants. Refer to Chapter 3 for further information. The best advice is to seek the employee with the highest and most appropriate credentials.

REFERENCES

1. Fullner, W: Complying with the State Law Against Discrimination in Employment. Association of Washington Business in cooperation with the Washington State Human Rights Commission, Washington.
2. All about OSHA, rev ed. United States Department of Labor, Washington, DC, 1982.

BIBLIOGRAPHY

Aiken, TD, and Catalono, JT: Legal, Ethical and Political Issues in Nursing. FA Davis, Philadelphia, 1994.
American Association of Medical Assistants: Health Care Law and Ethics. Chicago, 1996.
Hannon, S: The ins and outs of hiring new staff. Professional Medical Assistant 27(2):10, 1994.
Harlan, K: Conducting an employee evaluation. Professional Medical Assistant 27(3):4, 1994.
Lindh, W, et al: Comprehensive Medical Assisting, Clinical and Administrative. Delmar, New York, 1998.
Medical Office Manager: Considerations before firing an employee. Professional Medical Assistant 28(3):6, 1995.
Medical Office Manager: When you have to fire, there is a strategy. Professional Medical Assistant 28(4):8, 1995.
Parker, N: Interviewing, hiring and the ADA. Professional Medical Assistant 29(3):11, 1996.

Discussion Questions

1. In seeking an ambulatory health care employee, describe three places where you might look, and give the reasons for your selection.
2. When interviewing a candidate, a question is asked that the candidate refuses to answer, citing discrimination as a reason. What should you do?
3. The physician says to the assistant in the hall, "I'm tired of telling you how to do things and having you mess it up during an exam. Pick up your check at the end of the week and don't come back." How could this situation be prevented by using wise employment practices?
4. Under what conditions might office hours and the employee workweek be different? Why?
5. Your supervisor makes lewd remarks and obvious sexual advances. What will you do?

6. Dream a little. You have the "perfect" employee and want to show your appreciation. What might you do?

7. Describe the type of questions you would ask during an interview for potential employees.

8. You find the right candidate for the job and there are physical disabilities involved. What will you do?

9. For the position of clinical medical assistant, identify standards related to hazardous chemicals and bloodborne pathogens that must be in place.

A Cultural Perspective for Ambulatory Health Care

LEARNING OBJECTIVES

Upon successful completion of this chapter, you will be able to:

1. Discuss the impact of cultural influence on ambulatory health care.
2. Recall the components of cultural diversity.
3. Give an example of each component of cultural diversity.
4. Examine the concept of a new culture.
5. Identify any personal prejudice or bias and determine a strategy to address it.

*L*aws are obligatory rules for citizens to follow: otherwise, we face consequences. *Ethics*, however, are a set of standards that are voluntary. In the health care setting we adhere to laws governing medicine. Ethics exist in medicine also. Every health care setting will have its own culture of ethics. Each employee brings a set of ethics also. The blending of these different cultures is critical to quality client care.

What of cultural differences? Do we understand client's mores that differ from ours? Are we accepting of differences and similarities? Are we open minded? How will a better understanding of cultures help us be

---

CRITICAL THINKING EXERCISE

An Arab-American becomes belligerent when asked for a signature on a consent form. He has already agreed verbally to the procedure. The physician spends time with the client, discovering that once Arabs give their verbal agreement to a contract, they consider it binding and equal to a written consent.

more effective health care practitioners? In health care, cultural differences exist relative to age, gender, sexual orientation, ethnic background, educational preparation, life experiences, spiritual influences, role models and mentors, economics, and internal milieu.

■ COMPONENTS OF CULTURAL DIVERSITY

Ageism is any form of prejudice, bias, or discrimination that negatively targets the person on the basis of age. Children may be seen as property rather than trust; adolescents may be seen as moody people who seldom listen to others and are difficult to understand. Elders may be seen as hard of hearing, forgetful, opinionated, and set in their ways. The importance of age differs among cultures.

Gender issues are prejudices, biases, and discrimination based on sexual identity; whether you are a woman or man. It is sometimes used to refer to sex-based categories. For example, in some cultures men may be seen as dominant, athletic, mathematically inclined, and physically superior, whereas women may be seen as intuitive, caregivers, nurturers, and physically weak. Cultures may differ in their views of gender. Medical research in the United States has been predominantly on men. More studies are being done on women. In some cultures, women may take the lead in raising children, whereas in other cultures, the men may. In the United States some professions are predominantly male; however, that does not prohibit women from entering those fields.

Sexual orientation addresses issues of heterosexuals, gays, lesbians, bisexuals, and transvestites. In the United States, sexual orientation may be addressed by law in some states. However, widespread discrimination is common. A person's sexual orientation is important to health care not only in what pathology might be unique to the relationship, but also in the effects of illness on significant others.

Vignette 9

Two gay men in their 50s desire to adopt a child. One of the men has juvenile onset diabetes and is partially blind. These partners have sufficient financial resources. They are willing to accept a child with special needs.

Ethnic background is one's national heritage, race, tribe, clan, and language and may be related to geographic location. It is estimated that by 2050 Hispanics will be the largest ethnic group in the United States, yet how many citizens speak Spanish? The language barrier often implies that people have not yet learned to think in English; rather, they think in their native language. Family plays an important role in most cultures. Physical space, handshakes, and eye-to-eye contact vary with cultures. Some professionals may be respected more than others in some cultures.

CRITICAL THINKING EXERCISE

A 15-month-old Puerto Rican child enters the urgent care center with a history of persistent, productive cough, fever, sleeplessness, and congestion. The child is diagnosed with pneumonia and is to be hospitalized. The child is wearing a pretty bracelet with black and red stone beads. The mother explains that this bracelet is what protects the infant from the evil eye. Two hours later, a hospital nurse removes the bracelet. Discuss the implication.

Educational preparation is one's formal education, such as kindergarten through high school; some cultures have only 4 or 5 years of formal education. Some cultures have private education as the norm. Such differences may include private, public, or parochial education. People moving to the United States may come with a high level of skill and education recognized in their country but may be forced to take low-paying, menial jobs. Others may come with limited education and reap benefits from our education system. For others, language may prevent many from progressing in our education system.

Life experiences include death, divorce, disability, chronic illness, family crises, adoption, and surrogacy. Some may have siblings; others may be an only child; some may have been raised with extended family members. Such experiences shape how we adjust to life's challenges. A survivor of the Holocaust has seen and experienced persecution that few can comprehend. Veterans of wars experience events that shape their lives forever. They experience death and destruction few know. Divorce may be impossible in some cultures and simple to obtain in others. Disability may be seen as shameful, and some disabilities may be hidden. Other cultures give a person with disabilities great respect.

Spiritual influences may include any of the major religions or no religion. A person's belief system may be a separate and unique spiritual support system. Individuals with a belief in a supreme deity may be better prepared for surgery. They tend to "let another take charge." Some individuals are more ready for death and tend to accept it more easily because of their religious beliefs. Sometimes, too, people may view illness or disease as a "punishment" because of their religious views. People may see their religion as an explanation for health problems.

Role models and *mentors* may be family members, teachers, famous persons, pacifists, or warriors. Role models and mentors may differ within cultures; however, the way health care was role modeled is often the way one will use health care. For example, if health care is seen as a right by parents, children often will expect the same or more.

Economic influences stem from resources available, wealth and its distribution; the developing world versus industrial or informational affluence; dictatorship versus democracy. Individuals who do not have the economic resources to pay for their health care may do without. It may be difficult for people who come from a socialist health care system to adjust to a democracy. The third-party payer idea is an economic consideration. Some people may be able to pay cash and receive the care needed, whereas in other countries, it would be impossible to receive such services. In preventive medicine, we require inoculations, whereas in underdeveloped countries, people die from diseases these inoculations can prevent.

Values are morals or standards that are acceptable and practical in a culture. The value of life versus the value of death is a standard set by a culture. Values are determined by culture, family, religious beliefs, school, friends, and mentors. They are shaped by life experiences. Values are difficult to modify.

Internal milieu is what people cannot see, but it affects one's daily life. Many of the influences addressed previously affect one's internal milieu and how one reacts to life. A person can be diabetic with a chronic heart condition or have low self-esteem, but this may not be obvious. A person's internal milieu will affect how he or she approaches health care.

Cultural differences exist. Every standard and influence is culture bound. What is "right" in one culture may be considered "wrong" in another. We feel most comfortable in our own culture working within our own values. Rather than accentuate cultural differences, how can we learn to complement? Our culture is one among many. It has no special status. We need to develop a knowledge base and acceptance for differences in cultural mores and standards.

■ ESTABLISHING A NEW CULTURE IN AMBULATORY HEALTH CARE

Every exchange with a client is a cross-cultural one. Each person brings to that exchange a diverse background, experience, education, age, gender, race, ethnic origin, physical ability, religious belief, and sexual orientation. Developing another culture, if that is what it might be called, where there is mutual respect, acceptance, and an environment conducive to teamwork among clients, physicians, other health care providers, and ambulatory health care personnel must be the goal. Health care providers must recognize that the failure to accept such diversity among clients or the inability to embrace one's own differences becomes a barrier to client-physician communication and quality health care.

Entering into a new culture of mutual respect, acceptance, and teamwork does not require total agreement with another person's differences; it requires only acceptance of those persons for who they are and for what they believe. One must be nonjudgmental. It means seeing each person with a "clean and open slate," not one that has been tainted by one's own prejudice and bias. For example, we do not have to alter or change our sexual orientation in order to respect and accept a differing sexual orientation. We only must be able to see each person as a unique and special human being who has a right to quality health care and equal treatment.

Such a culture demands that each of us become more accepting and inclusive in our interactions with others. It requires that we become informed and knowledgeable of others' cultures. If several clients are Spanish speaking, learn Spanish so that at times you may converse in their language. Not only do you gain their respect, but you learn how hard it is to think in a second language.

To challenge your thinking further, consider the following scenario.

A male caregiver who is about 6 feet, 3 inches, and 250 pounds brings a 4-year-old boy into the clinic. It appears obvious that the child has been struck several times. While the physician is attending to the child's injuries, the very nervous male caregiver paces to the receptionist's desk, leans over, and says, "My God, what have I done? I did not mean to hit him so hard!" Your response might be, "Get out of my face, you SOB; the police will take care of you!" Or it might be, "How could a brute like you hit a child so small?" Or struggling to be therapeutic, remembering that the abuser is also a victim, and trying to accept this person, obviously distraught and upset, as another human being of equal value, you might reply, "As hard as this is for me, you've taken the first step in realizing your mistake. We're treating the boy now. Please just have a seat, try to remain calm, and I'll have the physician speak with you as soon as she's finished." Identify the conflicting values expressed.

In another scenario, examine the following:

> A middle-aged man comes out of the examination room and stops
> to make a follow-up appointment. You notice the tears in his eyes
> and ask how you can help. He sobs, "Not only must I go home
> and tell my wife I've been leading a life as a bisexual, I must also
> tell her I'm positive for HIV." You can respond by saying, "You
> play with fire, you're going to get burned. I pity your wife." Or,
> "Personally, I'd never go home. I'd drive my car off a cliff." Or
> again you can strive to put your prejudices and biases aside and
> respond, "How difficult this must be for you. I am sorry. Would it
> help if you asked your wife to come talk with us or to make an ap-
> pointment with the physician? What can I do for you?"

Consider a far different scenario.

> Your physician is treating a woman of Chinese ancestry. She is
> elderly and has been in this country only a few years. She is of-
> ten temperamental and angers easily. She tells you as she waves
> the prescription paper in your face, "No make me take this! Dr.
> Chin's herbs much better—much cheaper, too!" You can say,
> "You crazy old lady; just go see your Dr. Chin. Don't bother us
> any more. Insurance won't pay for him anyway!" Recalling
> your knowledge of the Chinese culture, and the importance of
> herbal medication, you can say, "You feel like Dr. Chin's herbs
> really help more? Did you share that with the physician? It may
> be OK to take both the herbal medicine and the prescription.
> Let's ask the physician just to be safe. We want you to get well."

Examine each prejudice or bias you hold. On what assumptions is it
based? Do those assumptions have any merit? Ask someone whose
judgment you value to assist you in this examination. Recall someone with whom you have great differences. Can you foster the kind
of respect and acceptance of that person to enable you to see him or
her as a human being with equal merit rather than as a person with
whom you disagree?

▮▮▮ SUMMARY

As we move into the section on bioethical issues, your culture and your
belief system will be challenged. In each situation, strive to remain as free
of prejudice as possible, thus allowing open examination of all sides of an
issue. Consider the following quotes:

"The real act of discovery consists not in finding new lands, but in seeing with new eyes." Marcel Proust

"A new idea is first condemned as ridiculous and then dismissed as trivial, until finally, it becomes what everybody knows." William James

BIBLIOGRAPHY

Calloway, K: Bioethical issues confronting the African American Community. Bioethics Forum 11(2):31, 1995.

Gregory, DR: Modern medicine in a multicultural setting. Bioethics Forum 11(2): 9, 1995.

Hamilton, J: Multicultural health care requires adjustments by doctors and patients. Can Med Assoc J 155(5):585, 1996.

Heide, J: Sheila and Nick and the world. Bioethics Forum 9(3):2, 1993.

Heide, J: Aunt Jewell and Sammie. Midwest Medical Ethics 6(2–3), 1990.

LaPuma, J: Cultural diversity in medicine and medical ethics: What are the key questions? Bioethics Forum 11(2):3, 1995.

McNair, D: In a different voice: technology, culture, post-modern bioethics. Bioethics Forum 11(2):35, 1995.

Pachter, LM: Puerto Rican health beliefs and practices: Exploring the boundaries between ethnomedicine and biomedicine. Bioethics Forum 11(2):15, 1995.

Rachels, J: The Elements of Moral Philosophy, ed 2. McGraw-Hill, New York, 1993.

Sample, T: Where's Will Rogers when we need him most? Bioethics Forum 11(2): 22, 1995.

Tamparo, CD, and Lindh, WQ: Therapeutic Communications for Allied Health Professionals. Delmar, Albany, NY, 1992.

Discussion Questions

1. *In each of the scenarios, what would be your response? Is your response accepting and nonjudgmental?*

2. *Interview two persons who are of a different culture than your own. Ask them how they access health care. What is the influence of the family unit? Who makes health care decisions?*

3. *Recall a time when you personally have been discriminated against in the health care setting because of your culture.*

4. *What role models and mentors have influenced your choice of health care?*

5. *Identify the largest ethnic minority in your geographic location. How are the health needs of this group addressed? What do you know about this group's culture?*

6. *What are the laws in your state addressing discriminatory actions related to sexual orientation?*

chapter 12

Allocation of Scarce Medical Resources

LEARNING OBJECTIVES

Upon successful completion of this chapter, you will be able to:

1. Define the term *macroallocation of scarce resources.*
2. Describe how decisions are made at the macroallocation level.
3. Define the term *microallocation of scarce resources.*
4. Describe how decisions are made at the microallocation level.
5. Describe both systems of selection.

DEFINITIONS

Apgar score. System of scoring an infant's physical condition 1 minute and 5 minutes after birth. Heart rate, respiration, muscle tone, response to stimuli, and color are measured. Maximum score is 10; those with low scores require immediate attention if they are to survive.

Bioethics. Morals or ethics connected with biology or medicine.

Diagnosis related groups (DRGs). Categorization of medical services to standardize prospective medical care.

Macroallocation. System in which distribution decisions are made by large bodies of individuals, usually Congress, health systems agencies, state legislatures, and health insurance companies.

Microallocation. System in which distribution decisions are made by small groups or individuals, such as hospital staff and physicians.

You are employed by a team of transplant surgeons in a major city when a call comes from a hospital that donor organs are available. The wheels move quickly to determine proper matches among the clinic's clients. Your physicians discover that two equally needy clients are waiting for the donor liver. One is an 18-month-old infant whose first liver transplant is being rejected. The other possible recipient is a 7-year-old recently diagnosed with liver failure. How is a decision made?

A young boy in a rural area of the country dies in a hospital after an automobile accident. Your physician, on emergency call at the hospital when the ambulance brings in the client, works feverishly for more than an hour, but the boy dies. Your physician relates to you the next morning the feeling of hopelessness of knowing the boy's life might have been saved if a neurosurgeon and more sophisticated equipment had been accessible to the hospital. How is it that geographic location may dictate who lives and who dies?

The family at 913 Twelfth Street will be saved from financial ruin because medicare will help defray the costs of their young son's kidney dialysis. The family at 909 Twelfth Street may suffer great financial stress because of increasing medical bills for the treatment of their daughter's juvenile onset diabetes mellitus, which has left her blind and nephrotic. How does our government determine that one medical problem warrants financial assistance and another does not?

When a 58-year-old employee, Sam, loses his job because his company is downsizing, he is unable to maintain his health insurance premiums for more than 6 months. He also finds it impossible to find any employment with similar pay and benefits. His wife, receiving care for cancer, is now left without insurance. Sam paid more than $60,000 of his money for his wife's care before her death, just 9 months after the health care coverage was lost. Sam is nearly bankrupt.

It is estimated that 60 million Americans will be without health insurance by the year 2000. Today, many are employed by companies who do not offer health care for employees. Many more are underinsured and, like Sam, would quickly go bankrupt if a medical catastrophe strikes. Do Americans have a right to basic health care?

A large portion of Americans without adequate health care are children. Prenatal care is an unaffordable luxury for the uninsured. Often, adequate care is unavailable even after infants are born. The elderly are increasingly having difficulties obtaining adequate health care. Medicare, with its increasing costs and decreasing coverage, is inadequate. Without a quality medicare supplement program, the elderly, like the nation's children, will go without. What value do we place on human life in our country when basic health care is not available to those who need it most?

With the ever-changing health care climate and the increased managed care contracts, health professionals in all facets of the industry, ambulatory as well as inpatient, are required to do more with less.

Hospitals and acute care centers have radically altered their delivery system of health care. For example, a surgical nurse with 10 years of experience may be moved to the role of circulating nurse, and a surgical technician with only 9 months of recent training will actually assist the surgeon. The circulating nurse is removed from the actual operation yet is ultimately responsible for the supplies and equipment in the room and documenting any incidents that might occur. Responsibility and accountability issues are shifting toward cost containment. In ambulatory health care physicians will seek the best person to fit the particular required skills. For instance, a medical assistant with both administrative and clinical experience is more appropriate in ambulatory care than a nurse. In addition, some services such as billing and transcription may be contracted by outside entities.

> These changes pose economic, ethical, and political questions.
>
> The economic question is, "How can scarce resources be allocated in light of the costs required and still satisfy human needs or desires?"
>
> The ethical questions are, "Is medical care a right or a privilege?" and "How will these scarce resources be justly and fairly distributed?"
>
> The political questions are, "Who will pay for basic health care?" and "Who decides what kind of benefit package everyone should receive?"

Health professionals, researchers, and members of nearly all academic disciplines have been formally discussing such issues for more than a decade. For discussion, it is easier to define the problem in terms of **macroallocation** and **microallocation** of scarce resources.

▅▅ MACROALLOCATION AND MICROALLOCATION

Allocation decisions deal with how much shall be expended for medical resources and how these resources are to be distributed. Macroallocation decisions are made by larger bodies, such as Congress, health systems agencies, state legislatures, health organizations, private foundations, and health insurance companies. For example, Congress determined that medicare should provide medical care for the client with chronic renal disease. No other chronic disease is specifically named in the medicare program. Macroallocation decisions also are evident when determinations are made regarding funding of medical research. How much should be allotted for cancer research, for preventive medicine, or for expensive equipment? The health insurance industry largely determines the "reasonable and customary" charges in medical care and therefore what will and will not be covered by health insurance premiums. Additionally, Congress has instituted a prospective payment system that reflects macroallocation called **diagnosis related groups (DRGs),** which categorize clients' conditions and identify them by number. Payment is made on the basis of a predetermined rate or average cost.

Microallocation decisions are made on an individual basis, usually by local hospital policy and doctors, concerning who shall obtain the resources available. Decisions at the microallocation level cut deeper into the conscience, because such decisions are personally closer to each of us. Examples requiring these decisions include hemodialysis machines and organs donated for transplantation. Who is allowed to occupy that one available bed in intensive care? Does the medicaid client receive the same care as the local VIP? Does a 60-year-old medicaid client have an equal chance at the kidney transplant as the foreign visitor who has cash to pay for the procedure? Who gets the flu shots when there is not enough vaccine for all those at risk?

▬▬ THE INFLUENCE OF POLITICS, ECONOMICS, AND ETHICS ON HEALTH CARE

States also enter into the political arena of macroallocation. For example, in 1989 Oregon passed the first program for rationing health care in the United States. The Oregon legislature created the Health Services Commission, which, after holding discussions in many public forums, presented a prioritized list of health services they believed warranted diagnosis and treatment. Illnesses below a certain number were not covered either because it was believed the persons would get well on their own or treatment would be futile. The Oregon Health Plan extends medicaid eligibility to all state residents with incomes below the federal poverty level; establishes a high-risk insurance pool for people refused health coverage because of preexisting health conditions; and addresses small businesses by offering them options to provide their employees with the ability to change jobs without losing their health insurance coverage. Other states are considering similar legislation. Some say the Oregon legislation is long overdue; others see the plan as an example of government controlling health care. In either instance, the plan does provide for treatable health care coverage, however limited, to all residents of the state. Only time will address its effectiveness, efficiency, quality, and cost.

With advancing medical technology and the increased choices in health care options, we have moved affordable health care outside of the reach of most consumers. Employers find it increasingly difficult to include a health care benefits package for employees. Purchasing health care insurance without a group is exorbitant. A family of four purchasing a health insurance policy with a high deductible can cost as much as $4500 per year. The American Medical Association fought long and hard to prevent government health care reform, fearing the loss of control in decision making. That control, however, has been compromised by the increasing stipulations of health insurance carriers and managed care contracts. The insurance companies fear they will be responsible for more services than premiums allow. Businesses continue to want to offer good health benefits to attract and to retain employees but understand that they cannot pass on those increases to customers and their workers indefinitely.

Whether the issue is macroallocation or microallocation, the problem is how best to maximize the health of the population with available resources.

◼ SYSTEMS FOR DECISION MAKING

How are the criteria established that attempt to answer such questions of allocation? Two prominent systems have arisen. The first system identifies three possible selection processes. The second system identifies five principles for a fair selection process. An outline of the two systems follows:

System I

1. Combination criteria system. Those who satisfy the most criteria ought to receive treatment. Such criteria might include the following:
   a. Capacity to benefit from treatment without complications
   b. Ability to contribute financially or experimentally as a research subject
   c. Age and life expectancy
   d. Past and potential future contributions of the client to society
2. Random selection system. This system is more like "first come, first served," or a simple chance selection or drawing of lots.
3. No-treatment system. This system is based on the premise that if all cannot be treated, treatment should be given to none.[1]

System II

Decisions should be made on the following bases:

1. To everyone an equal share
2. To everyone according to their individual needs
3. To everyone according to their individual efforts
4. To everyone according to their contributions to society
5. To everyone according to their abilities and merits[2]

■■■ HOW WOULD YOU DECIDE?

To enable you to appreciate more fully the difficulties in making choices related to the allocation of scarce medical resources and to assist you in establishing a criterion for selection, the following cases are given for you to ponder.

Example 1

You must make a decision regarding who will be allowed to enter the hospital. There are three clients; only two can enter because the remaining beds are full.

1. Determine the criteria from which you will make your selection.
2. Put the chosen criteria in writing and be prepared to support them.
3. Select the two clients from the following list. Justify your choice.

The cases are (1) a 55-year-old swimmer who has a heart attack at the local pool; (2) a 23-year-old woman ready to deliver her first child, whose attending physician suspects complications; and (3) a 9-year-old comatose accident victim with undetermined injuries.

Example 2

You have just given birth to a 20 oz infant of 6 months' gestation. The **Apgar score** is −2. The infant cannot suck and has no muscle tone, no gag, and no reflux. There is a need to protect the brain and the nervous center. The attending physician approaches you and the infant's father with the news that the only chance of survival is to transport the infant to a neonatal center in the nearest city, 200 miles away from home.

What is your response? The infant's father's? What problems do you foresee? What are the legal implications of your decision?

After discussing the situation, consider the following circumstances 6 months later. You made the decision to send the infant to the neonatal center. After 2 weeks, your medical bill was well over $100,000. You have only enough money to add to your medical insurance to cover a normal labor and delivery. It appears that the infant will be unable to come home for several weeks, if ever. The infant has now been diagnosed with the following problems: cerebral palsy; blindness; hydrocephalus, which has been alleviated with a shunt in the brain; and seizures.

What choices are available to you and the infant's father now? Who is responsible for the increasing hospital bill? Is medical care a right or a privilege under these circumstances? Who makes the decisions involved in this case?

At this point, it should be obvious that no established criteria provide clear-cut solutions to the aforementioned cases. None would be easy to follow. Factors other than those mentioned in the two systems will also influence decisions. They include personal ethics, personal preferences, religion, geographic location, legal requirements, and the political climate. Many problems and few solutions are evident when considering how and to whom scarce medical resources should be allocated.

Allocation of scarce medical resources is a complex issue of **bioethics,** but it is one the allied health professional cannot ignore because it presents itself frequently.

REFERENCES

1. Beauchamp, TL, and Walters, L: Contemporary Issues in Bioethics, ed 4. Wadsworth, Belmont, Calif, 1994.
2. Ibid.

BIBLIOGRAPHY

American Medical Association, Council on Ethical and Judicial Affairs, Code of Medical Ethics: Current Opinions with Annotations, 1996–1997 Edition. Chicago, 1996, pp 5–6.
Findlay, S: Experimental health plan makes its debut. USA Today, Friday, January 10, 1997, p 2A.
Zubler, NN, and Nimmons, D: Ethics on Call. Harmony Books, New York, 1992.

Discussion Questions

1. *Consider each of the examples at the beginning of the chapter and answer the following questions:*
   a. *At what level (macroallocation or microallocation) is a decision made?*
   b. *Can one of the selection systems be applied?*
2. *On what basis do you decide who gets the last open slot of the physician's appointment book? What system of selection is followed?*
3. *Two clients desperately need the use of one remaining hemodialysis machine. One is aged and a medicaid client. The other is a young college student who has full health insurance benefits. Who decides? Support your answer.*
4. *What suggestions do you have to make health care available to all? How would your plan be funded?*

5. *Form groups of three or more individuals to discuss Example 1. Consider the same circumstances. Consensus is necessary on your selection system and on the two clients to be admitted. What problems are encountered?*

chapter

13 *Genetic Engineering*

LEARNING OBJECTIVES

Upon successful completion of this chapter, you will be able to:

1. Name at least six diseases that can be detected by genetic testing.
2. Compare voluntary and mandatory genetic screening.
3. Describe three tests used for genetic testing.
4. Recall two indicators for amniocentesis and two possible outcomes.
5. Review the legal and ethical implications of sterilization.
6. Describe the Human Genome Project.
7. Define the term *gene therapy.*
8. Define *artificial insemination by husband* (AIH) and *artificial insemination by donor* (AID).
9. Identify circumstances that may warrant AIH and AID.
10. Describe in vitro fertilization and list its advantages and disadvantages.
11. Describe gamete intrafallopian transfer (GIFT) and list its advantages and disadvantages.
12. Define *zygote intrafallopian transfer* (ZIFT) and when it is used.
13. Describe intracytoplasmic sperm injection (ICSI).
14. Define the term *surrogacy.*
15. Discuss at least two ethical and legal concerns in surrogacy.
16. State three guidelines for ambulatory health care employees concerning genetic engineering.

DEFINITIONS

Amniocentesis. Method of prenatal diagnosis in which a needle is used to withdraw fluid from the amniotic sac within the uterus of a pregnant woman; fluid tested for genetic anomalies.

Artificial insemination. Instrumental introduction of semen into the vagina, cervical canal, or uterus so that the woman may conceive.

Blastocyst. An early embryonic cluster of cells that attaches to the uterus wall and develops into the actual embryo.

Chorionic villus sampling (CVS). A method of genetic testing whereby a flexible catheter inserted through the vagina and cervix sucks out a tiny piece of chorionic villi tissue on the outermost layer of the amniotic sac.

Down syndrome. A variety of congenital moderate-to-severe mental retardation. It is marked by a sloping forehead, small ear canals, gray or very light yellow spots at the periphery of the iris, short broad hands with a single palmar crease, a flat nose or absent bridge, low-set ears, and generally dwarfed physique. Also called trisomy 21.

GIFT. Gamete intrafallopian transfer; method of fertilization whereby the egg is removed during ovulation and placed in a dish. Sperm is concentrated and both egg and sperm are injected into fallopian tubes.

Hemophilia. Hereditary disease characterized by poor clotting ability; occurs almost exclusively in men; there is no known cure; also called bleeder's disease.

Heterologous artificial insemination by donor. Injection of a donor's semen into the vagina, cervical canal, or uterus to induce conception.

Homologous artificial insemination by husband. Injection of the husband's semen into the vagina, cervical canal, or uterus to induce conception.

ICSI. Intracytoplasmic sperm injection, in which an injection of a single sperm cell into a single egg occurs.

In vitro fertilization. Fertilization that takes place in glass as in a test tube under laboratory conditions.

Laparoscope. An instrument for examining the abdominal or peritoneal cavity that uses a fiberoptic light source.

Phenylketonuria (PKU). Hereditary disease caused by an enzyme deficiency; requires immediately starting a special diet to prevent complications such as mental retardation.

Sickle cell anemia. Hereditary, chronic form of anemia, affecting principally people of Mediterranean and African ethnic origins.

Surrogate. Substitute; someone or something replacing another.

Tay-Sachs disease. Hereditary disease causing degeneration of the nervous system, mental and physical retardation, and blindness. No treatment is available; prognosis is poor with death usually occurring within the first 2 to 3 years of life. Occurs almost exclusively among people of Jewish descent.

Ultrasound. Sound waves of extremely high frequency used to examine structures inside the body for diagnostic purposes; produces an image or photograph of an organ or tissue.

ZIFT. Zygote intrafallopian transfer is an intermediary procedure between GIFT and in vitro fertilization in which eggs and sperm are combined in the laboratory; the zygotes are inserted into the fallopian tubes.

Scientific developments during the 20th century have given rise to moral and social issues of considerable complexity. Recent advancements in genetic engineering, testing, screening, and assisted conception enable us to make new choices regarding human procreation and the creation of a healthful society and raise legal and ethical concerns never before considered.

The federally funded Human Genome Project has the National Institute of Health and the Department of Energy striving toward mapping the human genome and identifying all its estimated 50,000 to 100,000 genes by the year 2005. The success of this project has the potential of enabling each of us to view our genetic inheritance and any predisposition to disease. Gene therapy would allow the introduction of genes into existing cells to prevent or cure a number of diseases.

In the past, married couples expected to have children. Some couples determined the number of children they would have; others trusted that they would be able to care for as many children as they produced. A childless couple considered adoption.

Today, many decide to remain childless, seek sterilization, and invest their energies elsewhere. Those who want a child, whether married or not, can choose assisted conception such as **artificial insemination, in vitro fertilization (IVF)**, gamete intrafallopian transfer (**GIFT**), zygote intrafallopian transfer (**ZIFT**), intracytoplasmic sperm injection (**ICSI**), or surrogacy.

▨ GENETIC SCREENING, TESTING, AND COUNSELING

More than 3500 to 4000 genetically related disorders have been identified. In some cases, genetic testing is helpful in treating a client's disorder. In others, no treatment or cure is possible even if genetic testing can detect the carriers of many disorders as well as the sufferers.

Genetic testing and screening had its beginnings as a voluntary measure to discover persons already suffering from a particular disease. An example is **phenylketonuria (PKU)**. The second development was the institution of mandatory testing. In most states, PKU testing is now mandatory for all newborns. Also, some states require that applicants for marriage licenses be tested for the presence of the sickle cell trait, and no states allow the marriage of first cousins. In the latest stage in the development of genetic testing, tests seek to detect the carriers as well as the sufferers of particular genetic diseases.

Today genetic testing is done for variety of reasons. It can be used for prospective parents who wish to assess the risks of having a child with some disabling condition. Genetic testing can be done in utero to examine the chromosomes in fetal tissue to detect **Down syndrome** or other genetic disorders. Testing can be used in the legal setting to identify the source of blood, semen, and other tissue samples to determine the paternity of a child, to be used in cases of rape, assault, or murder. In the workplace, genetic testing has been used to test for inherited diseases or for genetic tendencies for cancer in case an employee would be exposed to potential toxins.

Genetic testing is performed by obtaining a blood sample and laboratory analysis, which can cost between $200 and $2000 per test. Through genetic testing and screening, a number of genetic diseases can be predicted with a certain degree of probability. Such diseases are **hemophilia, Tay-Sachs disease, sickle cell anemia,** Down syndrome, and PKU. Genetic testing exists for the genes that cause or contribute to some breast, ovarian, and colon cancers; osteoporosis; Alzheimer's disease; and Huntington's disease. The accuracy of the tests varies. It is recommended that persons who wish genetic testing consult a qualified genetic counselor.

Chorionic villus sampling (CVS) is a test used to detect genetic defects as early as the ninth week of pregnancy. In CVS, a flexible catheter inserted through the vagina and cervix sucks out a tiny piece of chorionic villi tissue on the outermost layer of the amniotic sac. This test can detect chromosomal defects.

A procedure related to genetic testing that is more familiar to the ambulatory health care employee is **amniocentesis,** the removal of fluid from the amniotic cavity by needle puncture.

The physician takes a sample of fluid surrounding the fetus by inserting a sterile needle into the amniotic cavity and withdrawing a small amount of fluid. This fluid, containing fetal cells, is centrifuged to separate the cells from the fluid. The cells are then studied for genetic defects. The procedure is performed no earlier than at 14 weeks of gestation and is generally done between 16 and 18 weeks of gestation.

Ultrasound is used in conjunction with amniocentesis for placement of the needle. Ultrasound is used to examine structures inside the body, much the same as radiographs but with the advantage that the client is not submitted to harmful radiation. Ultrasound is sound waves of extremely high frequency inaudible to the human ear. It is comparable to sonar systems used by submarines to find underwater objects. Sound waves are bounced off an object, producing a photograph.

The most obvious purpose of such testing is to determine genetic diseases that would cause suffering or death to the offspring, as well as an emotional burden on the family. There are two clear indicators to health professionals for the need for amniocentesis. One is advanced maternal age (40 years of age or older), which greatly increases the risk of Down syndrome. The second is the pregnancy of a woman who has previously borne a child with a genetic disease. The outcome of the procedure also is twofold. One outcome informs prospective parents of the difficulty so they may be better prepared to face the problem at the time of birth and in the future. The second outcome is the practice of selective abortion.

Neither outcome is an easy solution to a genetic disease, especially because the woman already is well into pregnancy by the time the results of amniocentesis are known. Selective abortion at such a stage can be a traumatic experience. All kinds of questions face the client who discovers a genetic disease through amniocentesis: Can I or the child live with the disease, and for how long? How "normal" will our lives be? What financial obligations will this put on the family? How will siblings be affected? Do I have a right to choose an abortion? Does the child have a right to life only or a right to a healthy, normal existence free from pain, agony, and deformity? Who decides? On what basis is a decision made?

Through amniocentesis, the sex of the unborn child also can be determined. Although this may serve only as a convenience to parents planning for the birth, some geneticists warn that some parents may choose selective abortion on the basis of sex only. Previously, physicians were reluctant to comply with parental requests to selectively abort a fetus. Consider, however, the number of cultures and countries in our world that prefer male offspring to female offspring. Many such countries have declining female populations, contrary to what is known about population statistics.

Genetic counseling generally is voluntary. Its purpose is to provide information rather than to dictate decisions on reproduction. Its goals are to decrease the number of children suffering from birth defects and genetic diseases and to offer information to prospective parents. However, such counseling can discourage the birth of children carrying harmful genes. On the negative side, genetic testing is part of a medical record, and insurance companies may cancel coverage based on test results and employees could be banned from employment based on test results. Questions exist, such as, "Will prenatal testing increase the use of abortions?" "Should any testing be done before the age of consent?" "Do you really want to know if the news is bad?" "Will you take any action if the news is negative?"

To further illustrate genetic testing and screening, consider the following situations and the possible ethical and legal ramifications.

A 45-year-old mother of six is expecting. She requests amniocentesis to check for Down syndrome. In an adjacent examination room, a young woman experiencing her first pregnancy is also concerned about Down syndrome. Her sister is afflicted with the disease. Knowing the tendency can be familial, she also requests amniocentesis. Will the genetic counseling of each woman differ? Support your answer. Each woman asks you, "What would you do in my situation?"

A case study from the *Hastings Center Report*[1] tells of a 45-year-old woman who is told she has Huntington's chorea, a genetic disorder for which there is no treatment. The disease causes irreversible mental and motor deterioration. The problem is that anyone who inherits the gene will develop the disease and will transmit the disease to some of their offspring. Most clients will be asymptomatic until age 40, after their childbearing years. The client in this case study has three children, and three sisters and one brother, but refuses to tell anyone about her diagnosis. What responsibility does this client's doctor have? Does this client have a moral responsibility to tell her family?

Vignette 10

Parents of a minor and incompetent girl, K.M., petitioned through counsel to be appointed guardians of her person and her estate. They also wanted authorization to consent to her sterilization.

K.M. has an IQ of 40 with a mental age of 6 to 7 years. Her independent functioning is severely limited. K.M.'s neurologist testified that she would never be able to exercise responsible judgment in sexual matters or in caring for a child. K.M. expressed to a counselor that she did not want to have children, but she may have been parroting what she heard her parents say.

The court ruled that K.M. could be sterilized, and her parents were granted authorization. Authorization was withheld pending appeal.

Outcome: Reversed and remanded. The court was found in error for not appointing independent counsel for K.M. Juvenile Law, Case Summaries, re the Guardianship of K.M., No. 25941-5-1 (Division One), September 16, 1991.

STERILIZATION

Sterilization is not a new issue. With society's concern about birth control and overpopulation, sterilization has become the most popular form of birth control in the world. Individuals whose genetic testing indicates they are a carrier for serious disease may also consider sterilization.

Sterilization for women is called tubal ligation and involves cutting, tying, and clamping the fallopian tubes so the egg will not meet the sperm and pass into the uterus. Tubal ligations are performed abdominally or vaginally.

Sterilization for men is by vasectomy. The procedure requires a local anesthetic and a small bilateral incision into the scrotum. Each vas deferens is pulled out and ligated. Follow-up of this procedure is important to ensure that all of the sperm have been discharged before sterility occurs. Two consecutive sperm counts must prove negative before any other birth control methods should be discontinued.

Some clients and physicians argue that individuals should have control over their bodies and that they alone should decide whether sterilization should occur. There is a strong argument against sterilization for eugenic purposes, and many consider involuntary sterilization mutilation. The rights of spouses in any sterilization procedure may need to be considered because their procreation function is affected also. However, states have granted no privilege to spouses or partners. Arguments also have been made by the legal guardians of severely mentally retarded persons for eugenic or involuntary sterilization.

Another ethical issue to consider is whether sterilization is a valid method of contraception. Society must bear some burden for the attitudinal pressure against large families. Some countries place severe tax penalties on couples who have more than two children. Many countries are conscious of a severe population explosion. Sterilization as a form of contraception has increased in the United States.

As so often is the case, physicians and their clients have to make decisions on sterilization alone, with little assistance from the law or agreed-on ethical standards. Physicians will perform sterilization procedures, for any reason, completely within the mandate of state statutes and only after receiving written, informed consent from the individuals involved. Careful counseling should be given in all cases. Physicians should help clients understand that the procedure removes the possibility of having children. Particular care will be taken in sterilizations of young adults who are unmarried or who have no children.

▬▬ HUMAN GENOME PROJECT AND GENE THERAPY

Human Genome Project's goal is to analyze the structure of human DNA and determine the location of all human genes. It also will help in the better understanding and treating of many genetic diseases. Such mapping of the entire human genome will revolutionize medical care because all of us have potentially harmful genes that put offspring at risk or put people at risk for disease in adult years. This is known as gene therapy.

Testing for a gene that causes disease will make it possible to diagnose conditions even before some symptoms appear. Presymptomatic diagnosis opens the door to the possibility of preventing the symptoms from occurring. Such diagnosis makes it possible to identify the inheritance for a condition in a family. A family could now know the risk of recurrence in the offspring and also may be able to have information for any possible preventive measures.

Gene therapy is not without serious concerns, however. If genes are to be replaced in the ovum or sperm, the replacement gene would be passed on to the next generation. This could be beneficial or harmful. For example, two copies of the gene for sickle cell trait cause sickle cell disease. If you replace the two sickle cell genes with two normal genes, you also eliminate protection from malaria, which is provided by a single copy of the sickle cell. Also, to date, no avenue is available that permits efficient, effective, and stable transfer of genes directly into a client.

With all the good this genetic research promises, it also raises ethical and legal dilemmas. Some genetic tests do no more than tell persons that some day they will suffer from a dreadful and progressive disease. Genetic tests will force wrenching decisions to be made by parents who may choose to abort rather than give birth to a child carrying a gene for a lethal disease.

As research progresses through gene mapping, it also is possible to locate those genes that govern traits such as intelligence and appearance. At this point, technology might move from the genetic engineering for the correction of disease into social engineering for the creation of a "superior" race. Some are so fearful of this possibility that they believe all such genetic research should be ended now. Others believe that the new genetic age will create a society that is healthier and has a more pleasant lifestyle.

CRITICAL THINKING EXERCISE

In February 1997 the first successful mammalian cloning took place in Scotland when a sheep, "Dolly," was cloned. One week later in the United States, Oregon successfully produced genetically identical rhesus monkeys through nuclear transfer. In 1996 it took more than 150 attempts and $150,000 for a biotech company to successfully clone a calf named Gene. Gene already has two fellow clones.

ASSISTED CONCEPTION

Recent scientific and technologic innovations in assisted conception have caused us to rethink the concepts of family, parenthood, and human sexuality. The biologic concept of family considers those people who are genetically related to be a family. However, this does not include the broader cultural customs and kinships that define family. Culture and kinship have to do with family relationships and are more subjective. We can divorce ourselves from our culture, our customs, and our kinship, but we cannot divorce ourselves from our genetic family.

Our societal laws determine the definition of family. We have laws on adoption, artificial insemination, surrogacy, foster placement, custody arrangements, and removal of children from homes where they are neglected or abused. Assisted conception raises complex issues such as the right to privacy and the right to make childbearing decisions, the interpretation of existing statutes that may relate to assisted conception, public policies regarding termination of parental rights, and the role of financial compensation in assisted conception.

Because we as a society are generally uncomfortable with human sexuality, we struggle when faced with circumstances outside of what we have learned is "normal." We are continually challenged to accept and embrace a broader view of human sexuality and family.

Such radical changes in society have strained the family unit, the legal system, the health care team, and our values. Any health care professional, whether in an ambulatory care setting or a hospital, cannot adequately function without knowledge of these concerns and their legal and ethical implications.

Assisted conception is a reality. Artificial insemination, in vitro fertilization, GIFT, ZIFT, ICSI, and surrogacy have captured popular attention. The use of semen from either a husband or a donor; the fertilization of the ovum in the laboratory for later transplantation in the uterus, fallopian tubes, or peritoneum; and the use of frozen sperm and embryos and the services of a **surrogate** mother are recent developments that provide alternatives to traditional modes of procreation.

▓▓ ARTIFICIAL INSEMINATION

As many as 25 percent of the couples in the United States are unable to have children. For whatever reason, infertility seems to be on the increase. At the same time, the number of infants available for adoption has declined. One possible solution to the dilemma is artificial insemination.

Artificial insemination is not a difficult procedure. It is simply the mechanical injection of viable sperm into the vagina, cervical canal, or uterus. This method has been practiced for thousands of years by individuals who had a strong desire to have a child. Approximately 40,000 children are born by artificial insemination each year.

Artificial insemination is described as (1) **homologous artificial insemination by husband** or (2) **heterologous artificial insemination by donor.** Artificial insemination by husband (AIH) might be used when a husband's sperm vitality is too low or a wife's cervical mucus is too hostile to achieve conception. Semen collected and concentrated over a few days often can overcome a low sperm count or a sperm vitality problem. Artificial insemination by donor (AID) might be used when the partner is sterile or carries serious genetic defects. It has also been used by women who want to have children but who choose not to have sexual intercourse with men.

Obstetricians and gynecologists are asked about AIH and AID almost daily. Physicians in these specialties and their employees need to be able to discuss the topic with intelligence and understanding. Women are sometimes referred by their physician to fertility clinics and specialists, which are found in most major cities. Some physicians will practice AIH but not AID, usually for legal and sometimes for ethical reasons.

■■■ LEGAL AND ETHICAL IMPLICATIONS OF AIH AND AID

Physicians will want to exhaust all available fertility testing before recommending AIH. On determining to proceed with AIH, care must be taken to explain the procedure, its effectiveness, and any possible problems. Permission to perform the procedures should be in writing, with both husband and wife consenting. Confidentiality must be ensured.

Artificial insemination by donor presents problems separate from AIH. Using the semen of a donor other than the woman's husband raises some questions: Does the donor have any right to the child? What kind of screening should be used to determine an appropriate donor? Can the physician be held liable if careful screening is not adhered to? Is an act of adultery committed?

In the past few years, more states have begun to address these questions legally. For the most part, however, few state statutes deal with artificial insemination. Before performing AIH or AID, physicians need to be aware of their state's laws. States with no laws on the subject rely on physicians to act with reasonable care and to protect themselves and their clients in the process. In such states, persons seeking AID would also be wise to seek legal counsel regarding the legal protection and parentage of the offspring.

Physicians may want the signatures of all parties involved in artificial insemination. The state of Washington requires that these signatures and the date of insemination be filed with the Registrar of Vital Statistics, where the file is kept confidential and sealed similarly to adoption records. Such a procedure or one similar seems wise when considering the ramifications of records kept only by the physicians involved.

For married couples, counseling should be done to ascertain that both the husband and wife want AID. Some men find accepting a child of AID more difficult than accepting an adopted child. However, the opposite can be true. Some men can accept AID children completely as their own. That acceptance is important.

When the woman is single, physicians need only her signature. The written consent of the donor is required in all cases. The donor's signature is to release all claims of paternity. The donor should not know who is receiving his semen, nor should the woman know the donor's identity. A relative also should not be considered as a donor. For the most part, selection of an appropriate donor is the responsibility of the physician. If the donor is married, consent from his wife should be obtained because her marital interests are also affected; however, this is not a legal necessity.

Some fertility clinics have a number of donors who can be called to bring semen when asked and usually are paid a fee for their services. Other clinics may rely on some of their employees or medical students. Although there are only a few sperm banks in the United States, they provide another alternative for suitable sperm.

Physicians and clinics using the services of sperm donors must screen carefully and meticulously. Some considerations include a complete physical and psychologic examination, a sperm analysis, a genetic history, and appropriate blood tests, including the test for the acquired immunodeficiency syndrome (AIDS) virus. Some physicians prefer donors who have already fathered healthy children. Careful consideration is also given to selecting a donor who has physical characteristics similar to those of the husband or those desired by the woman.

If in-house staff are used as donors, the utmost care must be taken to ensure confidentiality for all involved. For example, an intern who is a donor for a large medical setting may discover, either accidentally or purposely, the identity of a woman receiving his sperm.

Using frozen sperm for insemination is practiced more commonly. During a 6-month quarantine, the sperm undergoes extensive testing for disorders and diseases, showing a negative result for testing three times every 2 months.

Some physicians who perform AID recommend that the woman seek another physician, if she becomes pregnant, for prenatal care and delivery. This precaution may prevent any unnecessary questions regarding paternity of the newborn and may be wise in states that have not addressed the issue.

There are some ethical questions to consider in the whole realm of artificial insemination. Does the concept of sexuality being tied to the ability to procreate have validity? In other words, some people believe they lose their sexuality if they are unable to procreate. Society places much emphasis on fertility, even though there are many adoptable children in need of loving parents. These children often are not infants, may be multiracial, and may have physical or psychologic difficulties. Would society's emphasis be better placed on the needs of such children?

Should artificial insemination be performed on married women only? Who should be a mother? According to some religions, AID is adultery. Is the child then illegitimate?

What occurs in states in which no statutes have been enacted? Who monitors physicians practicing AID? Who ensures that donors have been carefully screened? What becomes of the AID records, after the death of physicians or when their practices close? Who has the ethical responsibility to prevent the potential marriages of people who have the same father through AID?

Those ambulatory health care employees who do not wish to be involved in AIH or AID for legal, ethical, religious, or any other reason need not be. Client referral can be made to other physicians or clinics who do perform artificial insemination. Medical health care employees who prefer not to be involved with artificial insemination should make that preference known before employment.

Those professionals involved in artificial insemination ought to remember that both men and women may be uncomfortable with the knowledge that several members of the medical staff know of their fertility problems and that AIH or AID is being attempted. Medical office assistants may have to ask men to manually produce their semen and to explain to women how that semen will be deposited, usually on more than one occasion, in their cervix without sexual intercourse. Treating these individuals in a professional manner, especially with the recognition that this is not an occasion for slapstick humor, will alleviate clients' anxieties and encourage open communication.

Artificial insemination is a truly private decision and an extremely personal procedure. Tact and courtesy are essential at all times, and the confidentiality and privacy of those involved must be carefully protected.

██████ IN VITRO FERTILIZATION, GIFT, ZIFT, AND ICSI

The development in genetics of in vitro fertilization (literally, "fertilization in glass") is the process of fertilizing the ovum in a test tube or culture dish, allowing it to grow, and then implanting it in the uterus. This procedure has been accomplished successfully in several species of animals for many years, and animal breeders have been selectively altering their stock for a better breed. Successful test-tube fertilization and embryo transfer in humans was achieved in the early 1980s.

A benefit of in vitro fertilization is that it allows many women who are infertile because of blocked fallopian tubes or oviducts to bear children. This is done by removing the ovum from the potential mother and placing it in a dish containing blood serum and nutrients. Sperm is added. Once an egg is fertilized, it is then transferred to another dish where, for the next 3 to 6 days, it divides, creating a cluster of cells called a **blastocyst**. The blastocyst is placed in the uterus, where it attaches to the wall and development proceeds.

An alternative to in vitro fertilization is gamete intrafallopian transfer (GIFT). This procedure lets the egg and sperm unite in the woman's body instead of in a laboratory dish. In GIFT, the woman's reproductive system is stimulated with hormones to help her produce four or more eggs. The physician monitors the woman and during ovulation removes the eggs with a **laparoscope**. Sperm is extracted from the man and concentrated. The woman's eggs are put in a laboratory dish until they are mature; then they are loaded into a long catheter with air followed by the sperm solution. The catheter is threaded through the laparoscope to a fallopian tube and discharged. Generally, fertilization occurs in the woman, as does implantation.[2]

Gamete intrafallopian transfer has been used with women who do not completely ovulate, for those with endometriosis, and for couples with unexplained infertility. However, the woman has to have at least one open fallopian tube.

Zygote intrafallopian transfer, ZIFT, is an intermediary procedure between GIFT and in vitro fertilization. In this procedure, eggs and sperm are combined in the laboratory. If fertilization occurs, the zygotes are inserted into the fallopian tubes.

Intracytoplasmic sperm injection, ICSI, is injecting a single sperm cell into a single egg that is used when sperm are low in number or motility or when men have no live sperm in their semen as a result of vasectomy, chemotherapy, or a medical disorder. The fear in ISCI, thus far unfounded, is that the sperm may pass on more genetic defects than "normal sperm" would or that ICSI might preserve defective sperm cells.

It is possible to use frozen ova either before or after fertilization. Frozen immature eggs survive better than mature eggs, so the immature eggs have a better chance of surviving in the woman's body. This technique also permits genetic testing before fertilization.

In in vitro fertilization, GIFT, ZIFT, and ICSI donor egg and donor sperm may be used. Some medical centers offer lists of healthy young women who for a fee will provide eggs that can be fertilized in the laboratory and implanted in infertile women. The average cost is $10,000 for each attempt at a pregnancy with donated eggs. Sperm banks also are available; however, men are paid much less for each donation, approximately $40.

▉ LEGAL AND ETHICAL IMPLICATIONS OF ASSISTED CONCEPTION

Informed consent from all involved parties is extremely important in assisted conception. The primary role of the physician is to inform clients of all aspects of the process. Clients should be allowed to make all necessary decisions, and physicians should only be "enablers" of the process rather than the decision makers. All agreements should be in writing. The physician should certify the signatures of all involved.

Confidentiality is the second legal implication. Physicians and their employees must keep information in the strictest confidence at all times.

Discussing such an issue freely, even with the physician, is often difficult for clients. The possibility that any information might become available to a third party through an overheard telephone conversation or a mislaid medical record is intolerable both to the medical profession and to the clients. Care must be taken to preserve the dignity of all involved. Comments made by staff need to be pertinent, informative, helpful, and nonjudgmental.

CRITICAL THINKING EXERCISE

A postmenopausal woman in her early 60s is pregnant. She is one of about 100 or so such reported pregnancies worldwide. These women turn to reproductive technology. A common response to this situation is, "How disgusting! Think how old she'll be when the child graduates from high school!" On the other hand, if a 62-year-old man fathers a child, the comment most likely will be, "How virile and manly to consider that someone that age could father a child!"

Additional specific concerns, more ethical in nature, must be considered. For instance, in vitro fertilization and GIFT are expensive, ranging from $2000 to $5000 per attempt, and may cost as much as $10,000 if eggs are donated. These procedures are not covered by insurance and thus are more likely to be performed only for the affluent. Should this procedure be available to anyone whether or not they can afford it?

Many argue that in vitro fertilization and related procedures are unnatural and an attempt to "play God." Will the increase in assisted conception lead to a frozen embryo bank? Who are the legal parents of an infant born of assisted conception? Perhaps equally critical, what rights does the conceptus have? Will the procedure be used to select sex? Who decides?

SURROGATE MOTHERS

A surrogate mother is one who agrees to conceive a child by AID, carry it to term, and relinquish it to the sperm donor after birth. In this instance, the surrogate and the offspring are genetically related. A surrogate mother also may serve only as a "host" for a fertilized ovum contributed by another woman and man. After birth, the infant, who has no genetic link to the surrogate, is relinquished to the natural father and mother. Generally, a preconceptual contractual agreement dictates that the surrogate mother will relinquish all rights to the newborn. A fee is paid to the surrogate mother by the donor. Ordinarily, the donor also pays for all the expenses of the procedure. In 1994 surrogate mothers generally received $10,000.

▬ LEGAL AND ETHICAL IMPLICATIONS OF SURROGACY

One of the problems in establishing laws in this area is that we do not understand what the long-term effects of surrogacy will be; also, we cannot determine what, if any, may be the psychologic and social risks to the infant.

Surrogacy received national attention in 1987 when a surrogate mother in Newark, New Jersey, chose not to relinquish the infant she bore to the child's biologic father and his wife, who had contracted with the surrogate *(Stern v Whitehead)*. The courts ruled in favor of the biologic father and allowed his wife to adopt the infant. The decision was appealed to the New Jersey Supreme Court. In what became known as the "Baby M" case, the New Jersey Supreme Court ruled that the child's father, William Stern, could retain custody of the 22-month-old child but that Mary Beth Whitehead-Grould, the surrogate, maintained her rights as a parent.

In California, Crispina and Mark Calvert hired Anna Johnson to gestate an embryo composed of the Calverts' egg and sperm. The Calverts paid Johnson $10,000 and purchased life insurance for her during pregnancy. During the pregnancy, the Calvert–Johnson relationship soured, and Johnson requested her money earlier than agreed on. Before the delivery of the baby, both the Calverts and Johnsons brought suits, each side claiming parental rights. The Orange County Superior Court said that a "three-parent, two–natural mom situation" would confuse the child and "invites financial and emotional extortion." The court concluded that Johnson and "the child are genetic hereditary strangers." The judge compared the contract between the Calverts and Johnson to a common foster-care arrangement in that Johnson was "providing care, protection, and nurture during the period of time that the natural mother, Crispina Calvert, was unable to care for the child."

Obviously, the difficulty in surrogacy arises when the surrogate mother has to relinquish rights of the infant she bore. Some argue that it is similar to baby buying and baby selling. Others argue that without fees surrogate mothers would have little or no reason to offer their services. The New Jersey Supreme Court in the "Baby M" case stated that "baby selling potentially results in the exploitation of all parties involved" and that payment in a surrogacy contract is "illegal and perhaps criminal."

Finally, any time there is a contract, mistrust on the part of one or more parties is a possibility. All parties involved in surrogacy have to deal with questions of morality and of right or wrong. Significant legal issues include whether contractual arrangements between the parties are legally enforceable and what parental rights, if any, the participants have in the child. Some states with legislation on the issue have declared surrogacy invalid. Other states have no statutes.

Complex questions are asked: What is the meaning of family? Will lineage be disrupted? What if the parents are unfit? Which relationship takes precedence—that of the adoptive mother and child or that of the surrogate mother and child? What happens if the infant is deformed? Who decides?

As long as technology advances further and faster than the legal system can address these developments, ethical dilemmas will continue.

■ CONSIDERATIONS FOR AMBULATORY CARE EMPLOYEES

Genetic screening, testing, and counseling, sterilization, assisted conception, and gene therapy are delicate topics. For clients to be open and honest about their concerns, all employees involved must demonstrate a professional attitude. Confidentiality must be protected. Informed consent is especially important. Employees' personal views on these matters should be fully explored before seeking employment in a facility that actively participates in any procedure related to genetic engineering. Also, those personal views should not be made known to clients during or after the decision-making process. In the area of gene mapping and therapy expect to have the Human Genome Project suggest ethical and legal guidelines for its use before its completion.

In genetic engineering, knowledge of state statutes and recent court decisions is necessary to act within the law. When there is doubt, an attorney should be consulted.

REFERENCES

1. Lynch, A: The price of silence. *Hastings Cent Rep* 20(3):31, 1990.
2. Kolata, G: Egg donors raise ethical questions. New York Times, November 10, 1991, p A8.

BIBLIOGRAPHY

American Medical Association, Council on Ethical and Judicial Affairs, Code of Medical Ethics: Current Opinions with Annotations. Chicago, 1996, pp 19–29.
Ames, K: And donor makes three. Newsweek, September 20, 1991, pp 58–61.
Annas, GJ: Crazy making: Embryos and gestational mothers. *Hastings Cent Rep* 21(1):35, 1991.
Capron, AM: Whose child is this? *Hastings Cent Rep* 21(6):37, 1991.
Furrow, BR, et al: Health Law, Vol 2. West, St Paul, Minn, 1995, pp 520–545.
Grady, D: How to coax new life. Time 148(14):37, 1996.
Hotz, RL: Legacy of uncertainty. The Sun, November 10, 1991, p B1.
In brief: Held to a higher standard. *Hastings Cent Rep* 21(3):2, 1991.

Macklin, R: Artificial means of reproduction and our understanding of the family. *Hastings Cent Rep* 21(1):5, 1991.
McCabe, ERB: Medical genetics. JAMA 275(23):1, 1996.
Prenatal test reveals inherited retardation. The Sun, December 12, 1991, p A2.
Raeburn, P: Detection of fetal ills improved. News Journal, October 9, 1991, p A1.
Tinley, ST: Human Genome Project: Where Will It Take Us? National Institute on Deafness and Other Communication Disorders (NIDCD), Hereditary Hearing Impairment Resource Registry (HHIRR), Omaha, Nebr, 1996.

Discussion Questions

1. *Should genetic screening or testing be mandatory for any disease? Support your answer.*
2. *Why is informed consent essential for a sterilization procedure?*
3. *Should permission of a spouse be mandatory for sterilization?*
4. *Why does AID pose more of a problem, ethically and legally, than AIH?*
5. *Discuss how you might handle the medical records of individuals involved in AID if the Registrar of Vital Statistics is not interested in them.*
6. *A couple comes into the ambulatory health care setting for AID. They have determined that the husband's brother should be the donor and already have made arrangements with him. What counseling would you suggest?*
7. *Describe possible problems of in vitro fertilization.*
8. *Professor Joseph Fletcher, bioethicist and noted author, says, "It is unethical and morally wrong to deliberately or knowingly bring a diseased child into the world, or to turn a cold shoulder on prenatal tests. Never bring a baby into the world with anything more than minimally serious defects or disease." Discuss.*
9. *Paul Ramsey, professor of religion at Princeton University, says, "We cannot begin by bloodying ourselves with the killing of our own kind because they are defective in the womb, without also going into infanticide of similarly defective born infants." Discuss.*
10. *Katherine is a surrogate mother for a couple living 15 miles away. Katherine, near term of pregnancy, decides she does not want to relinquish the baby. What she does not know is that the prospective mother was killed in an auto accident 2 weeks ago. Who has the right to the child? How is a decision made?*
11. *What are the ethical concerns related to gene therapy?*
12. *Describe the positive implications of GIFT, ZIFT, and ICSI.*

14 *Abortion*

LEARNING OBJECTIVES

Upon successful completion of this chapter, you will be able to:

1. Define the terms *abortion* and *miscarriage*.
2. Describe the process of fetal development.
3. List five theories of when life begins.
4. Explain the methods of abortion.
5. Discuss the Supreme Court decisions on abortion from 1973 to the present.
6. Analyze three major ethical issues on abortion.
7. Describe the use of fetal tissue in research and transplantation.
8. Identify guidelines for abortion in ambulatory care.

DEFINITIONS

Conceptus. General term referring to any product of conception.

Eugenic abortions. Abortion performed because the fetus is severely deformed or damaged.

Infanticide. A type of homicide consisting of killing the newborn.

Mitosis. The process by which the cell splits into two new cells, each having the same number of chromosomes as the parent cell.

Ovum. The female germ cell.

Quickening. The first perceptible movement of the fetus in the uterus.

Spermatozoon. The male germ cell.

Therapeutic abortion. Abortion performed to preserve the life or health of the mother.

Zygote. The fertilized ovum; the cell produced by the union of gametes.

Abortion, the termination of pregnancy before the fetus is viable, is a highly emotional issue that elicits controversy no matter what the setting. Medically, the terms *abortion* and *miscarriage* both refer to the termination of pregnancy before the fetus is capable of survival outside the uterus.

FETAL DEVELOPMENT

Fertilization occurs when a **spermatozoon** (sperm cell) unites with an **ovum** (egg) within a few hours of sexual intercourse. Normally, this takes place in the fallopian tubes, after which the fertilized ovum, now called a **zygote,** begins its journey to the uterus (womb). The zygote begins a process of **mitosis** (cell division) during the approximately 3-day journey to the uterus. Mitosis continues while the zygote floats freely in the uterus and begins to attach itself to the uterine lining. The proper term for this attached ball of cells is a blastocyst.

The blastocyst continues development and attachment to the uterus until firmly implanted at the end of the second week. From the third week until the end of the eighth week, the blastocyst is called an embryo. During this time, organ systems begin to develop, and some features take on a human shape.

At approximately the eighth week, the embryo becomes known as a fetus and is marked by the beginning of brain activity. The term *fetus* is used until the time of birth, usually 9 months after fertilization. The 9-month period is generally divided into three segments, or trimesters. The first trimester is from fertilization to 3 months; the second trimester is from 3 to 6 months into the pregnancy; and the third trimester is from 6 to 9 months (Table 14–1).

WHEN DOES LIFE BEGIN?

Because most definitions of abortion refer to the viability of a fetus, it is important to define the term *viable. Taber's Cyclopedic Medical Dictionary*[1] defines it as "capable of living, as a newborn or a fetus that has reached a stage, usually 24 weeks or greater than 500 gm, that will permit it to live outside the uterus." Although not all experts agree, some sources put the time of viability at from 20 to 35 weeks.

Increasingly, however, there are instances when a fetus delivered before 20 weeks has survived. Medical technology has made tremendous advances in keeping premature infants alive, making it increasingly difficult to legally define viability. In underdeveloped countries, however, where there is little medical technology, the time of viability may surpass 35 weeks.

TABLE 14–1
Fetal Development

End of Approximate Month	Size and Weight	Representative Changes
1	$\frac{3}{16}$ in	Eyes, nose, and ears not yet visible. Backbone and vertebral canal form. Small buds that will develop into arms and legs form. Heart forms and starts beating.
2	$1\frac{1}{4}$ in $\frac{1}{30}$ oz	Ossification begins. Limbs become distinct as arms and legs. Digits are well formed. Major blood vessels form.
3	3 in 1 oz	Eyes almost fully developed but eyelids still fused; external ears present. Appendages are fully formed. Heartbeat can be detected. Body systems continue to develop.
4	$6\frac{1}{2}$–7 in 4 oz	Head large in proportion to rest of body. Face takes on human features, and hair appears on head. Many bones ossified and joints begin to form.
5	10–12 in $\frac{1}{2}$–1 lb	Head less disproportionate to rest of body. Fine hair covers body. Rapid development of body systems.
6	11–14 in $1\frac{1}{4}$–$1\frac{1}{2}$ lb	Head becomes even less disproportionate to rest of body. Eyelids separate and eyelashes form.
7	13–17 in $2\frac{1}{2}$–3 lb	Head and body more proportionate. Skin wrinkled and pink. Seven-month fetus (premature) is capable of survival.
8	$16\frac{1}{2}$–18 in $4\frac{1}{2}$–5 lb	Testes descend into scrotum. Bones of head are soft. Chances of survival are much greater at end of eighth month.
9	20 in 7–$7\frac{1}{2}$ lb	Additional subcutaneous fat accumulates. Nails extend to tips of fingers.

> Five possible considerations of when life begins are
> 1. at the time of conception
> 2. when the brain begins to function, usually at 8 to 12 weeks
> 3. at the time of **quickening,** 16 to 18 week
> 4. at the time of viability, from 20 to 35 weeks
> 5. at the time of birth

Some religious groups, including Roman Catholics, claim that life begins at conception because the blastocyst carries the genetic code for a new human being. The theory also is seen in the Chinese and Korean cultures, which count a child as 9 months or 1 year old at the time of birth.

Another determination for the beginning of life is at the time the brain begins to function. Proponents of this theory believe the fetus cannot be a human without a functioning brain. Because there is strong support for the idea that death occurs when the brain ceases to function, it may be logical to believe that life occurs when the brain begins to function.

Quickening has been determined by some to be the beginning of life. Aristotle believed that before quickening, the human fetus had only a vegetable or animal soul.[2] Another reason for this position perhaps is that women truly feel "life" at the time of quickening.

The idea that life begins when the fetus is viable or can live independently of the uterus is partly based on the premise that if the fetus indeed can live on its own, life has begun. More variation of time is allowed in this theory if you consider that viability may be sometime between 18 and 35 weeks.

Vignette 11

A married couple have five healthy daughters but want a son. The wife is pregnant and wants prenatal diagnosis solely to learn the sex of the fetus. If the diagnosis cannot be made, the wife wants to abort the fetus. Also, if the diagnosis shows the fetus to be female, she wants to abort the fetus. The husband believes that prenatal diagnosis to determine sex is wrong and does not want to consent to the testing. He convinces his wife to abort the fetus without knowing the sex. An abortion was performed, but the wife agonizes and wonders years later if she made the "right" decision.

Note: This vignette was derived from several case studies by Wertz, DC, and Fletcher, JC: Fatal knowledge? Prenatal diagnosis and sex selection. Hastings Cent Rep pp 25–26, May/June, 1989.

Those who believe that life begins only at the time of actual birth believe so because now the being can be seen, can be held, and is perceived as being fully human.

◼️◼️◼️ METHODS OF ABORTION

The method of abortion will depend to a great extent on the stage of the pregnancy. The descriptions given are from *It's Your Body* by Lauersen and Whitney.[3]

The morning-after pill, although not a method of abortion, is the earliest intervention of possible pregnancy. The theory is that high doses of estrogen over a few days prevent the fertilized egg from implanting in the uterine lining. The pills are taken for approximately 5 days and must be started within 72 hours of unprotected intercourse. Morning-after pills are often used in the case of rape or incest.

Mifepristone, formerly known as abortion pill and RU486, is available for use in France, China, Sweden, and Great Britain. Mifepristone, taken in pill form with a prostaglandin, "works by blocking the action of progesterone, which is crucial in order to sustain a pregnancy. Without progesterone the lining of the uterus breaks down and menstruation begins, expelling any fertilized egg."[4] It is most effective during the first 9 weeks of pregnancy. Mifepristone may be the preferred treatment because it is noninvasive, has no risk of infection, requires no anesthesia, is less expensive, and offers greater privacy to women. It can be used in the early stages of pregnancy. Mifepristone also shows promise in the treatment of progesterone-dependent breast cancers, meningioma, endometriosis, fibroid tumors, Cushing syndrome, and the human immunodeficiency virus. In September 1996 the Food and Drug Administration (FDA) found the drug "approvable" but requested that more information be provided to the FDA on manufacturing and labeling before its approval. Advances for Choice, a new privately held company, is likely to be identified as the US distributor of Mifepristone. At the time of publication, final approval has not been awarded by the FDA for the manufacture and distribution of this drug, but approval is anticipated.

The safest and quickest approved method of abortion, if a pregnancy test is positive and it is less than 7 weeks from the last menstruation, is called menstrual extraction, or miniabortion. In this procedure, a tube with a suction device is inserted through the cervix into the uterus (dilation is usually unnecessary). Within 1 to 2 minutes, the lining of the uterine wall and the **conceptus** are suctioned out. Cramping, nausea, and faintness may be experienced by a woman undergoing this procedure. It is commonly performed in the ambulatory health care setting.

To terminate pregnancy between the 7th and 12th weeks, a physician performs a suction abortion, or curettage. The procedure is similar to the miniabortion. In the ambulatory health care setting a local anesthetic is given, and the cervix is dilated to permit suction and scraping of the uterine lining. In a hospital, a general anesthetic is used. Cramping, nausea, and vomiting usually follow the procedure. The client can go home approximately 2 hours afterward.

These methods of abortion occur in the first trimester up to the 12th week of pregnancy. The period of 12 to 16 weeks affords few safe methods of abortion because the fetus is too large for a suction abortion and there is insufficient amniotic fluid for a saline injection. During this time, two possible methods are multiple vaginal or intramuscular administration of prostaglandins, which encourage expulsion of the conceptus within 10 to 15 hours. Dilation and the removal of the conceptus by suction and forceps is followed by curettage. These methods are relatively new and lengthy procedures that require close observation. Research is likely soon to produce other prostaglandin methods for the 12- to 16-week period of gestation that will be less complex and easier to administer.

Saline injection is performed between the 16th and 24th weeks of gestation. The procedure involves withdrawing between 50 and 200 ml of amniotic fluid through a needle and syringe. Approximately 200 ml of saline solution is then injected slowly into the remaining amniotic fluid. This procedure brings about normal labor and delivery of the fetus within 18 to 20 hours. The same procedure is used to instill prostaglandin into the amniotic sac, except only a small amount of amniotic fluid is removed. The results are the same. These procedures can be performed only in a hospital and require a stay of $1\frac{1}{2}$ to 3 days.

In a very few cases, a hysterotomy is performed to remove the fetus surgically. This is considered major surgery, requiring hospitalization and a longer period of recuperation than any other method. It is usually performed only in the case of uterine abnormalities.

Generally, the later an abortion of any type is performed, the greater the risk. Psychological and physiological difficulties can and may accompany any method of abortion. When pregnancy is to be terminated, for any reason, only qualified physicians and appropriate facilities should be used. Women are advised to seek professional help as soon as possible for their own safety and well-being.

◼◼◼ ABORTION AND THE LAW

In 1880 no abortion laws existed in the United States. When a woman wanted an abortion, she received it. By 1900 nearly every state had laws prohibiting abortion and treating it as a criminal offense. Nearly a century later, federal and state abortion laws still exist, but they tend to allow more freedom than those in the early 1900s.

One of the monumental decisions affecting a change of all abortion laws was the 1973 US Supreme Court *Roe v Wade* decision. Jane Roe (a pseudonym) was a single, pregnant woman who took action against Henry Wade, the District Attorney of Dallas County, in 1970. Roe pleaded the Fourteenth Amendment and her "right to privacy," claiming the Texas anti-abortion statute unconstitutional. As a result, 3 years later the Supreme Court held that during the first trimester, pregnant women have a constitutional right to abortions, and the state has no vested interest in regulating them at that time. During the second trimester, the state may regulate abortion and insist on reasonable standards of medical practice if an abortion is to be performed. During the third trimester, the state interests override pregnant women's rights to abortions, and the state may "proscribe abortion except when necessary to preserve the health or life of the mother."[5]

Although this court decision did "favor" Roe, many unanswered questions resulted. For example, when is the fetus viable? Is the fetus "property" of the bearer? Does the woman alone have the right, or do husbands, partners, or parents have rights? Can state and federal funding be required for abortions? Virtually every state statute on abortion was invalidated, either partly or totally, by *Roe v Wade*. The public responded to their legislators, who, in turn, reacted through legislation. Some state statutes set facility requirements where abortions were to be performed; others addressed filing of detailed reports on abortions performed, what consultation needs to be done before an abortion, and other such requirements.[6]

Another US Supreme Court decision in 1976 changed state abortion statutes. The court ruled, on constitutional grounds, that spousal and parental consent is not necessary for an abortion. Currently courts tend not to differentiate between minor and adult pregnant women.[7] Absolute parental consent may force pregnant minors to seek criminal or self-induced abortions. A 1978 US Supreme Court decision held that a state may not constitutionally legislate a blanket, unreviewable power of parents to veto their daughter's abortion.

In the 1977 *Doe v Bolton* case, the Supreme Court struck down four preabortion procedural requirements: (1) residency, (2) performance of the abortion in a hospital accredited by the Joint Commission on Accreditation of Hospitals (JCAH), (3) approval by a committee of the hospital's medical staff, and (4) consultations.[8] It also had a "conscience clause" stating that physicians and medical employees could refuse to participate in abortions without being discriminated against.

In June 1977 three related cases, *Real v Doe, Maher v Doe,* and *Poelker v Doe,* resulted in Supreme Court decisions affecting abortion laws. The ruling stated that "the states have neither a constitutional nor a statutory obligation under Medicaid to provide non-therapeutic abortions for indigent women or access to public facilities for the performance of such abortions."[9]

In 1983 the Supreme Court reaffirmed the *Roe v Wade* decision when it heard *Akron v Akron Center for Reproductive Health, Inc.* In Akron, three physicians and the center brought suit against the city challenging the constitutionality of city provisions that regulated abortion performance. The city had passed an ordinance requiring that (1) second-trimester abortions be performed in hospitals, (2) specific information be given by physicians to patients undergoing abortion, (3) there be a 24-hour waiting period between consent and performance of the abortion, and (4) there be specific procedures about how physicians were to dispose of the fetal remains. The case was appealed to the U.S. Supreme Court, which found all provisions unconstitutional except for the hospitalization requirement for second-trimester abortions.

Justice Sandra Day O'Connor contended in her dissent in the Akron case that "the Roe framework, then, is clearly on a collision course with itself. As the medical risks of various abortion procedures decrease, the point at which the State may regulate for reasons of maternal health is moved forward to actual childbirth. As medical science becomes better able to provide for the separate existence of the fetus, the point of viability is moved further back toward conception."[10]

In a similar case in 1986, the US Supreme Court again reaffirmed *Roe v Wade.* In *Thornburgh v American College of Obstetricians and Gynecologists,* the Supreme Court ruled against the following issues: informed consent and printed information that would have required a physician to provide information 24 hours before the abortion related to available medical assistance benefits; the father's liability for assistance; a description of alternatives to abortion; possible detrimental effects not foreseeable; and medical risks of the abortion, as well as of carrying the child to full term.

Additionally, the Supreme Court struck down a ruling that would have required physicians to determine whether the fetus was viable and to report to the State Department of Health specific information normally considered private. This information would have included such items as the woman's age, race, number of pregnancies, marital status, and date of last menses. This information was to be open for public inspection without the woman's name.

Third, the Supreme Court ruled against physician involvement in postviability care for the child and the requirement for a second physician at postviability abortions.

In 1991 the US Supreme Court upheld a ban on abortion counseling at federally funded clinics. This ban affects approximately 4000 clinics serving 4.5 million women, mostly with low incomes. The result is that these clinics cannot mention abortion as an option. Some clinics receiving federal funds have chosen to do without the funding so that abortions still can be presented as an option. Many observers think that this ban and the greater issue of abortion will be fought in the political world rather than in the courts.

In July 1992 the US Supreme Court, in *Planned Parenthood v Casey,* ruled that Pennsylvania's requirement that spouses be notified before abortion was an "undue burden." The US Supreme Court will probably be asked to consider laws from Guam, Utah, and Louisiana that have banned the majority of abortions in their jurisdictions. Lawyers say to uphold these laws, the court would have to overturn *Roe v Wade* or make it "an empty shell."

CRITICAL THINKING EXERCISE

A woman on welfare may be denied abortion if seeking federal funding. Discuss this in light of the Constitution.

Legal challenges are currently in process, and more Supreme Court decisions are expected. The majority of abortion questions arise over the Fourteenth Amendment and the equal protection clause. Every citizen of the United States has "equal protection of the law" and shall not be discriminated against. This includes abortion. The parties are testing the courts on these constitutional issues. For example, is it discriminatory for a woman who has money and insurance coverage to receive an abortion but a woman who is poor and relies on welfare to be denied an abortion? Will this withstand the scrutiny of the court on the issue of discrimination? Is there a rational basis for discrimination in the case of an unmarried woman versus a married woman seeking abortions? Can a state require a married woman to obtain her husband's consent? Can a state require a physician to inform the parents of a juvenile who is undergoing an abortion?

A recent report summed up the uniquely complex intersection of individual rights, public interest, and advances in medical technology:

Social response to women's reproductive abilities typically has made their bodies part of the public domain in a way that men's are not. Modern medicine, right in step with this tradition, has made women's wombs even more thoroughly public—its technology renders them open to view, and its science tells us with growing precision how the actions of pregnant women affect the health of fetuses.[11]

The abortion issue and the abortion law are in a state of flux. Radical changes have occurred in the past 100 years. Who can predict what the next 100 years will bring? The political climate, moral attitudes, advances in medical technology, and impact of current abortion laws will influence the future of abortion.

ETHICS AND ABORTION

Three major ethical issues surface in a discussion on abortion. Considering these issues separately is being neither honest nor realistic. The issues are as follows:

1. Are there any reasons to justify abortions?
2. Are current laws regarding abortions consistent, fair, and just?
3. Are abortions an appropriate method of birth control?

Are There Any Reasons to Justify Abortions?

To answer "Yes" with no restrictions implies that abortions should be performed on demand and at any time during the pregnancy as long as the procedure is still safe. The viability of the fetus or the circumstances are not issues to consider. The issue is a woman's right to make a decision on whether, if, or when an abortion is to be performed. The pregnant woman's right is higher than any other. The issue is one of freedom and human rights. Proponents of this theory may be called pro-choice.

To answer "No" without any other consideration is to believe that abortion for any reason is murder. The consideration here is that the fetus is innocent, weak, and helpless, and its right to life should be protected at all costs. These individuals often believe that to allow abortion is to also condone **infanticide.** The rights of the fetus and newborn are paramount to the rights of any others. Proponents of this theory may be called pro-life.

There are individuals who stand somewhere in the middle. These are the advocates who believe that abortion is permissible to save the life of the mother (**therapeutic abortion**). This situation receives support from pro-choice individuals. The second situation making abortion permissible and receiving support is in the case of rape or incest. For some, the circumstances determine whether an abortion is performed or the fetus is allowed to survive. This premise considers the rights of both mother and fetus and the rights of any others who may be involved. Most likely, pro-choice individuals also consider the question of when life begins.

One may expect that the church offers a solution to the question of when life begins. In discussing ethical questions, actions of the church are often considered. But there is no consensus or agreement here that settles the issue. A few religious groups propose that abortions be performed only when necessary to save the mother's life. Some religious groups determine a time or establish viability of the fetus for performing abortions. All make an attempt to understand the pain and trauma associated with any decision on abortion.

CRITICAL THINKING EXERCISE

The father of an unborn has no legal rights in an abortion decision. However, if a welfare mother gives birth, names the father, and it is verified, the father will be forced to give financial child support.

Are Current Laws Regarding Abortions Consistent, Fair, and Just?

This second ethical question may be somewhat easier to answer than the first; however, there is no general agreement on a response here either.

As was discussed earlier, laws were consistent in the early 1900s—abortions were illegal. The issue came into full public view in 1973 with the *Roe v Wade* Supreme Court decision. Statutes then changed, and abortion became legal.

These statutes are inconsistent, however. The Supreme Court's intentionally vague ruling has left the states to interpret and regulate abortions. Much variation remains. There is little agreement on the viability of the fetus or what regulations, if any, are established for physicians and facilities. Therefore abortions that are legal in one state may be illegal in another.

The consideration of how abortions are to be funded is even more complex. The 1977 Supreme Court ruling that said states were not required to fund abortions for the indigent woman raises the question of fairness and justice in following the law. Essentially, this ruling has the force of denying an abortion to a woman unable to pay. The right to choose becomes hinged on the ability to pay. This, in effect, denies personal freedom in a free society that has guaranteed equality under the Fourteenth Amendment. The other side of the coin means that opponents of abortion will pay through their taxes in medicaid funding for those who choose abortion. Persons who object on this basis also must weigh the costs of a funded abortion against the pregnancy, delivery, and welfare costs of the mother and child.

According to the National Abortion Federation Internet Web Page, the cost of an early, outpatient abortion is about $200 to $400, whereas a later abortion might be $400 to $700. The National Family Planning and Reproductive Health Association in 1994 found that for every dollar spent by the government to pay for abortions for poor women who want them, about $4 is saved in public welfare and medical costs resulting from unintended births. Another financial consideration to be faced is the care, support, and institutionalization of severely deformed infants born if **eugenic abortions** are not allowed. One cannot hold that abortions are morally wrong and therefore should not be funded without being an advocate of health facilities that provide care for babies who require institutionalization.

Are Abortions Appropriate Methods of Birth Control?

The third ethical issue is the most recent issue and has the least information available for discussion. The two highest incidences of "abortions on demand" come from individuals who do not practice birth control because it is not available to them or because it is not convenient. The two groups range in age from 20 to 24 and from 15 to 19, respectively, are white, and are unmarried.

Without debating contraception, for one reason or another contraception was not practiced, and the pregnant women sought an abortion. This is further complicated by data indicating that some of the same women return a second or third time for abortions.

Is something amiss in the moral standards of our society that may cause or force a teenager to seek an abortion because she felt too guilty or ashamed to practice contraception? It has taken the fear of AIDS to bring our country to the point where sexuality (and more specifically, contraception) is a topic of national discussion and concern. Yet, for many, perhaps most, this topic is still one of considerable discomfort.

Perhaps the problem has developed because easily accessible abortions have encouraged sex without responsibility. Is information about abortions more readily available than information on contraception? Is sex education, whether in the home or school, adequate? Are parents intentional and realistic about teaching morals? Bringing a new human being into the world is a privilege and a responsibility, and it should not be left to accident as a result of exploitation, fear, or ignorance.

There is no quick, easy response to this dilemma, and the problem is growing. Repeated abortions may affect future pregnancies. The psychologic impact of convenience abortions is not yet fully understood. As a society, we have not yet felt the full force of the medical or ethical ramifications of this issue.

Of interest is the fact that the number of American women obtaining legal abortions has fallen to its lowest level in nearly two decades. the US Centers for Disease Control and Prevention (CDC) reports that the number of legal abortions among women ages 15 to 44 decreased to 21 per 1000 in 1994, the lowest rate since 1976.[12]

■■■ FETAL TISSUE RESEARCH AND TRANSPLANTATION

Tissue from aborted fetuses has been used in research studies for transplant therapy benefiting people with such diseases as diabetes, Parkinson's disease, and Tay-Sachs disease. Fetal tissue cells are considered preferable to other tissue because they are less vulnerable to rejection. Should fetal tissue be used for research and for transplant? Will it save lives? Will it destroy lives? Abortion opponents believe the latter and fear that using fetal tissue from aborted fetuses could lead to fetal tissue clinics for harvesting and fetal tissue banks for storage. Advocates believe that fetal tissue is the best hope for millions of Americans who are diseased. Transplants could cure diseases and save lives.

In 1988 the Reagan administration banned federal funding for research using tissue from aborted fetuses. Bush continued the ban; however, in late 1991 the House of Representatives passed a bill to restore federal funding for human fetal tissue research. The bill requires women who are willing to donate fetal tissue to certify in writing that they did not have the abortion with the intent to donate. Such certificates would be kept on file by the researchers and would be available for government audit.

Controversy exists. Once a woman has consented to an abortion, will she be approached by researchers for donation of fetal tissue? Will people who have diseases or their families put pressure on politicians to allow fetal tissue research to continue? Does asking women to certify in writing that the abortion is not for the sole purpose of donation interfere with their privacy? Does the bill protect the confidentiality of the women? As with the abortion issue itself, research on fetal tissue causes ethical dilemmas.

AMBULATORY HEALTH CARE PROTOCOL

Physicians and employees must understand their own feelings on abortion. Those feelings should be based on medical fact. Their personal understanding of abortion will enable them to make a decision before their actual involvement. Legally, employees and physicians cannot be forced to participate in abortions against their wishes. The right to refuse, however, does not authorize the right to judge.

Physicians and employees who participate in abortions are wise to adhere to the following:

1. Participate only within the law.
2. Provide medical knowledge to clients on the stages of pregnancy, viability of the fetus, and methods of abortion.
3. Obtain written, informed consent.
4. Provide counseling as indicated by the situation.
5. Refer as necessary.
6. Keep records confidential.
7. Seek legal counsel when indicated.
8. Be understanding and compassionate.

REFERENCES

1. Taber's Cyclopedic Medical Dictionary, ed 18. FA Davis, Philadelphia, 1997, p 2084.
2. Thompson, JB, and Thompson, HO: Ethics in Nursing. Macmillan, New York, 1981, p 75.
3. Lauersen, N, and Whitney, S: It's Your Body: A Woman's Guide to Gynecology. Berkley Books, New York, 1983, pp 282–300.
4. Rosenthal, MS: The Gynecological Sourcebook. Lowell House, Los Angeles, 1995, pp 328–329.
5. Furrow, BR, et al: Health Law. West, St Paul, Minn, 1995, pp 480–502.
6. Rhodes, AM, and Miller, RD: Nursing and the Law, ed 4. Aspen Systems Corporation, Rockville, Md, 1984, p 289.
7. Ibid, pp 289–290.
8. Galvin, JH, and Mendelsohn, E: The Legal Status of Women. In The Book of the States, 1980–1981. The Council of State Governments, p 39.
9. Ibid.
10. Callahan, D: How technology is reframing the abortion debate. Hastings Cent Rep 16:34, 1986.
11. Nelson, JL: The maternal-fetal dyad: Exploring the two-patient obstetric model. Hastings Cent Rep 22(1):13, 1992.
12. The Seattle Times: Abortion rate down. Friday, January 3, 1997, p A8.

BIBLIOGRAPHY

The Washington Post: Feb 13, 1997. Settlement clears way for sale of mifepristone.
Harkness, C: The Infertility Book: A Comprehensive Medical and Emotional Guide. Celestial Arts, Berkeley, Calif, 1992.
Rosenthal, MS: The Fertility Sourcebook. Contemporary Books, Chicago, 1995.
The Feminist Majority Foundation: Reports on mifepristone, fertility control. Arlington, Va.
USA Today: Mifepristone makes giant step forward in FDA approval process. Sept 19, 1996.

Discussion Questions

1. *In your own words, describe the process that occurs in fetal development.*
2. *Prepare a 2-minute speech for laypersons on the methods of abortion.*
3. *As an antiabortionist, how would you respond to these problems?*
   a. *Pregnancies and resultant births from rape or incest*
   b. *Unwanted children*
   c. *Infants with severe birth defects*

4. As a pro-choice individual, how would you respond to these problems?
   a. Abortion as contraception
   b. A live aborted fetus
   c. The right to life versus the right to freedom

5. Where might you refer a patient for abortion counseling in your community?

6. Outline the Supreme Court abortion rulings in the 1970s, 1980s, and 1990s.

7. Under what conditions is an abortion legal in your state?

8. Your physician begins to perform miniabortions and you are not sure you can participate. What will you do?

Acquired Immunodeficiency Syndrome

chapter 15

LEARNING OBJECTIVES

Upon successful completion of this chapter, you will be able to:

1. Describe human immunodeficiency virus (HIV) infection and acquired immunodeficiency syndrome (AIDS) disease process.
2. Name at least one opportunistic disease of AIDS clients.
3. Discuss at least four ethical implications related to HIV infection.
4. Identify at least three legal implications related to HIV infection.
5. Discuss the implications for ambulatory health care employees related to AIDS.

DEFINITIONS

CD4. A protein on the surface of the cells that normally helps the body's immune system combat disease.

Opportunistic infection. An infection, usually fungal or bacterial, that results from a defective immune system that cannot defend against pathogens normally found in the environment.

Pneumocystis carinii. The organism that causes pneumocystis pneumonia, a lung disease characterized by slight fever and difficulty in breathing; this disease is often seen in persons with AIDS (Figs. 15–1 to 15–3).

▬▬ THE DISEASE PROCESS

The acquired immunodeficiency syndrome (AIDS), the disease that follows infection with the human immunodeficiency virus (HIV), is the world's number-one health concern. During the 15 years of HIV/AIDS reporting in the United States through June 1996, 548,102 men, women, and children with AIDS have been reported to the Centers for Disease Control and Prevention (CDC), and 343,000 have died. Statistics from

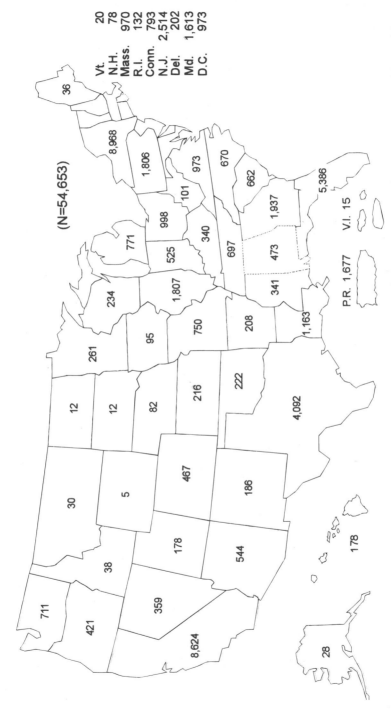

Figure 15–1. Male adult/adolescent AIDS cases reported in 1996, United States. (From the HIV/AIDS Surveillance Report, vol 8, no 12.)

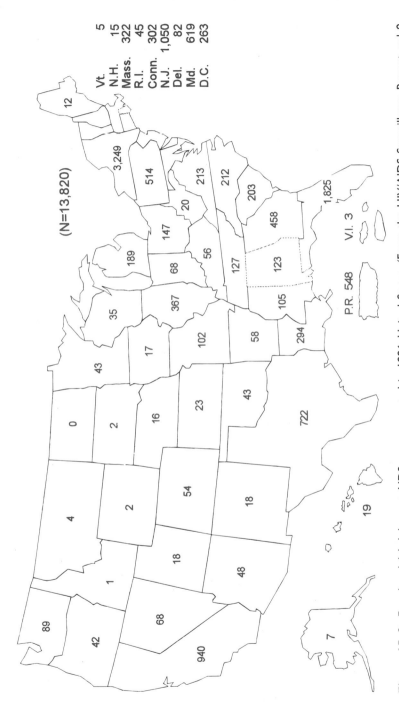

(N=13,820)

Vt.	5
N.H.	15
Mass.	322
R.I.	45
Conn.	302
N.J.	1,050
Del.	82
Md.	619
D.C.	263

Figure 15–2. Female adult/adolescent AIDS cases reported in 1996, United States. (From the HIV/AIDS Surveillance Report, vol 8, no 12.)

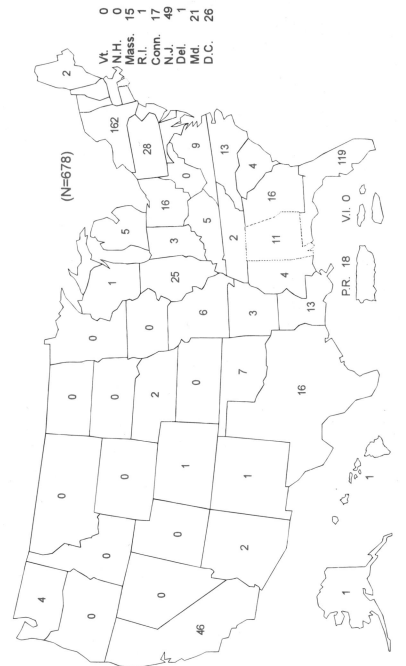

Figure 15–3. Pediatric AIDS cases reported in 1996, United States. (From the HIV/AIDS Surveillance Report, vol 8, no 12.)

1995 report that an estimated 20 million people living outside industrialized countries are infected with the AIDS virus.[1]

The transmission of the virus generally is through the blood, through semen during a sexual encounter when the tissue lining breaks, through the exchange of blood when a needle used by an infected person (usually a person with a drug dependency) is used by someone else, or through a blood transfusion from an infected person. This last mode of transmission has greatly lessened in incidence because of a test that detects the AIDS virus in donated blood.

An AIDS antibody test has been developed to detect if a person has been exposed to the AIDS virus. A positive test means that the person is infectious and can pass the virus to others. However, a positive test does not indicate whether the person has or will develop AIDS. Individuals testing positive for the virus may remain symptomless for quite some time.

Human immunodeficiency virus destroys white blood cells. Because the missing white blood cells are part of the immune system and are needed to protect the body from infections and certain cancers, individuals can eventually develop enough serious infections or cancer to cause death. Acquired immunodeficiency syndrome reduces the ability to fight infections, causing individuals to become progressively vulnerable to many other illnesses. The defenses of anyone with AIDS eventually collapse; death usually results from complications of one or more **opportunistic infections** such as *Pneumocystis carinii.*

According to the CDC, the HIV disease progression can be measured even before symptoms occur. When HIV establishes itself in the body, the number of **CD4** lymphocytes begins to decline. If the number falls below 300, individuals are at heightened risk for one or more opportunistic infections. If the CD4 cell number drops below 200, an individual is said to have AIDS.

As we learn more about HIV infection and how it affects the body, we learn more about the diseases that are more likely to exhibit themselves in HIV clients. With that knowledge, medical professionals are better able to treat clients earlier and more effectively. In the past, some persons with AIDS were misdiagnosed and received treatment for only the opportunistic infection.

The more common and specific opportunistic infections include *Pneumocystis carinii* pneumonia, *Toxoplasma gondii, Mycobacterium tuberculosis, Mycobacterium avium intracellulare,* cytomegalovirus, fungal infections, bacterial infections, herpes simplex virus, varicella-zoster virus, *Cryptosporidium,* and *Microsporidium.*

Toxoplasma gondii is a parasite that causes toxoplasmic encephalities, the most common cause of brain lesions in people with HIV infection. Dementia caused by HIV infection of the brain is the most common neurologic complication. It may be reported as HIV encephalitis or subacute encephalopathy, but the term *AIDS dementia complex (ADC)* is most commonly used.

With an already weakened immune system, HIV-positive persons must avoid exposure to *Mycobacterium tuberculosis* and *Mycobacterium avium intracellulare,* which are common infections in HIV-positive people.

Cytomegalovirus is a common cause of eye disease (retinitis) in people with HIV infection. It also can cause disease of the gastrointestinal tract, nervous system, and other organs.

Fungal infections are common but not life threatening for HIV-positive persons. The fungal infections are easy to diagnose and respond quickly to treatment.

People with HIV infections are more likely to develop respiratory infections, including pneumonia, which are usually caused by common bacteria and treated as any bacterial infection.

Herpes simplex virus is a common infection. It is controversial whether its treatment prolongs survival in people with HIV infection.

Varicella zoster virus can reactivate in adults with HIV, causing shingles.

Cryptosporidium and *Microsporidium* are parasites that can cause chronic and severe diarrhea in HIV-positive persons with low cell counts.

Treatment is symptomatic. Antibiotics, radiation, chemotherapy, and surgery may prolong life. In 1987 azidothymidine (AZT) was the only approved antiviral drug for adults with AIDS. In 1991 dideoxyinosine (ddI [Videx]) was approved. Dideoxyinosine is used for persons in advanced stages of infection with AIDS who do not respond to or cannot tolerate AZT. Both drugs slow the progression of AIDS but do not cure the disease. In December 1995 the FDA approved a new drug called saquinavir,

Vignette 12

A 33-year-old man works in a local food-handling plant in a small northern Minnesota town of 3000. The plant employs approximately 14 people and sells wholesale to the public for the larger surrounding community. The man begins to lose weight, feel weak, and develop coldlike symptoms, which soon cause him to miss days of work. His employer visits him at home to find he is living with another man and has been diagnosed with acquired immunodeficiency syndrome (AIDS). The man is able to work but is weaker.

Before long, the community knows his diagnosis, and the food-handling plant loses a significant number of buyers. The employee with AIDS continues to work at the plant when he is physically able. Finally, someone attempts arson on the plant. The arson was an attempt to let the employer know that the community member does not want a person with AIDS working in the plant.

which is a protease inhibitor. Doctors began to order a potent cocktail of saquinavir, AZT, and another powerful drug called 3-TC, a chemical cousin of AZT. Experiments are continuing on many other drugs, but it is too early to know for certain how successful treatment will be. Also of note is that the drug combinations cost tens of thousands of dollars a year, an expense even the well insured will have difficulty with.[2]

Statistics constantly change but are included here to inform the reader about the disease and the populations most at risk. Currently in the United States among adults and adolescents, three HIV exposure groups account for nearly all the cases of AIDS: men who have sex with men, intravenous drug abusers, and heterosexual contacts of persons in high-risk groups or persons who have HIV/AIDS. The number of persons with AIDS among ethnic minorities is increasing; those most often affected are blacks and Hispanics.[3]

ETHICAL IMPLICATIONS

The spread of infectious disease always has caused alarm in a country that takes pride in its health care, but never in this century has the fear been so great as in the face of the growing AIDS epidemic. This fear, coupled with the fact that there is no known cure, makes discussion of the disease's ethical implications difficult. However, another matter may be at the root of all the ethical concerns regarding AIDS. Much of society views homosexuality and drug abuse as unnatural, immoral, or illegal. This attitude makes it extremely difficult to view the illness free of prejudice. However, health care workers have a professional responsibility to provide nonjudgmental health care. Persons with AIDS are people with a disease who need care and treatment.

Unlike the other bioethical issues discussed in this book, individual choice may not be so clear in this matter as in others. One can choose not to have an abortion, choose not to be a surrogate mother, choose not to be involved in artificial insemination, and choose not to commit active euthanasia. Individuals may, however, contract AIDS through no choice of their own. For example, as of June 1996, there were 7296 cases of pediatric AIDS, 90 percent resulting from transmission of mother to child.[3] Others have been infected with the disease through the transfusion of infected blood before the development of a test that indicates the presence of the AIDS virus.

Some of the most pressing ethical questions concern the rights and responsibilities of infected persons. Do they have a right to treatment? If so, by whom? Do they have a right to employment? Do they have a right to privacy? Do they have a right to public education? Can they be excluded from medical or life insurance benefits? Will the government subsidize medical care for persons with AIDS? Do persons with AIDS have a responsibility to inform the public of their disease?

CRITICAL THINKING EXERCISES

You go in for elective surgery, and your surgeon says, "It is my practice to inform clients that I am HIV positive." Do you have surgery?

A client goes into a medical center for treatment and informs the physician that she is HIV positive. Does the physician care for the client?

The cost of medicine for the treatment of AIDS is extremely high. Many persons with AIDS find themselves with no health care insurance or in a plan that is withdrawn when costs soar.

There are great ethical problems over educating the public regarding the disease. Can we talk about "safer sex" in the media? The public seems comfortable with explicit sex in the media, but safer sex has caused a great deal of consternation, and only the most daring have entered the arena. How, too, can the public be adequately informed when there are still many unknowns regarding the disease? Although it is most commonly transmitted through blood and semen, some people are convinced that any contact is dangerous. What risks can individuals take and still remain safe?

Persons with AIDS probably have more to fear from the public than the public has to fear from those whose immune systems are so impaired they must fear contracting other diseases from the public. In some instances, society has been brutal to persons with AIDS. Homes of victims have been destroyed and individuals driven out of their communities, fired from their jobs, and refused medical treatment. Such actions encourage persons with AIDS to remain silent about the disease. How can we keep the public and persons with AIDS safe without harming either group or neglecting health care? One thing seems certain: There are no easy answers.

LEGAL IMPLICATIONS

Legal ramifications of the AIDS issue are closely aligned with the rights and responsibilities of persons with AIDS, the public, and health care providers. Surely these rights will be tested. For a person with HIV to knowingly infect another person may be a criminal offense in some areas. There is currently much discussion regarding mandatory testing for AIDS. It is most apt to start with the application for a marriage license. If AIDS testing becomes mandatory, how will the privacy of those involved be protected? Can employers require AIDS testing of their employees? All employees, or only certain employees whose jobs are at seemingly higher risk than others? What constitutes "higher risk"? Might quarantine be mandated? If so, under what circumstances? Can health care providers be forced to provide medical care to persons with AIDS? Must persons with AIDS inform their teachers or school nurses of their medical condition? Some states have enacted legislation in these areas, but it is certainly subject to change in the near future.

MANAGED CARE

In the whole arena of managed care, who is responsible for the long-term health care costs for HIV-infected persons who are likely to lose insurance coverage and employment possibilities?

Insurance companies generally are requiring HIV testing for those persons seeking life insurance policies of $100,000 or more. Also, applicants for individual health insurance policies may be asked if they have tested positive for HIV. If so, they may be denied health coverage. Some insurance applicants may be asked specific questions leading to HIV testing, such as "Have you had an unusual weight loss?" Some recommend that if an employee is leaving one place of employment and joining another that the old health insurance coverage be kept until the new plan pays for preexisting health conditions. A request for a change in health insurance coverage may trigger HIV testing.

Taken to the far end of the spectrum is Cuba's plan to stop the spread of AIDS. The government mandates that everyone old enough to be sexually active is tested for HIV. Every person found to carry HIV, symptomless or not, is quarantined in one of seven sanitariums where they are under guard.[4]

Congress, CDC, and the American Medical Association are pressuring HIV-infected health care workers to restrict their practice to noninvasive procedures or to disclose their status to clients. Yet the *Hastings Center Report*[5] tells of a survey in San Francisco that is showing a reverse effect. For example, of the HIV-infected doctors surveyed, 67 percent said they "avoided seeking treatment or submitting insurance claims through their place of employment because they feared job discrimination and loss of privacy." Also, "57 percent of those who did not know for sure whether they were infected expressed reluctance to be tested, preferring uncertainty to knowledge that could cost them their jobs."

Through June 1997, the number of U.S. health care workers with documented and possibly occupationally acquired AIDS/HIV infection was reported to be 114. See Table 15–1. However, health officials emphasize that it is very unlikely that a client will get AIDS from a health care professional. It is far more likely that physicians and other health care professionals performing invasive procedures on AIDS-infected persons will get the virus from those individuals.

Two federal statutes, Section 504 of the Rehabilitation Act of 1973 and the Americans with Disabilities Act (ADA), prohibit discrimination against persons who are disabled, which includes health care workers with infections of communicable diseases such as HIV and AIDS. Several HIV and AIDS cases have been tried under these statutes. Although HIV and AIDS are not specifically referred to in the statutes, HIV infection is substantially limiting, allowing it to be included. Under the ADA, the health care employer is required to make "reasonable accommodations" for health care workers who are HIV positive. Such accommodations have to be made that would reduce or eliminate any direct threat by the health care worker to clients; however, the ADA does not require that the health care worker be excluded from invasive procedures.

The Rehabilitation Act has been central to suits alleging discrimination by health care facilities against persons with AIDS. Facilities must provide "reasonable accommodations" for clients seeking treatment and care for HIV and AIDS. One cannot refuse to care for such clients. In fact, according to the American Medical Association's Code of Medical Ethics, physicians cannot refuse to treat clients with AIDS when their condition is within the physician's realm of competence. Physicians who are known to be seropositive should not engage in any activity that creates transmission of the disease to others.

▄▄ IMPLICATIONS FOR AMBULATORY HEALTH CARE EMPLOYEES

Ambulatory health care employees must be knowledgeable about the AIDS disease process, especially how the disease is transmitted, both for their own safety and for their client's protection. Health professionals should practice the Communicable Disease Center's universal precautions at all times. Such measures address aseptic clinical procedures on all clients whether or not they are known to be HIV positive (Table 15–1).

Precautionary measures must be taken. Most larger cities have special AIDS clinics that offer current information and referral systems for both health care workers and persons with AIDS. Persons affected by the AIDS virus have the same rights as anyone suffering a disease. They have the right to the same privacy as any others in the ambulatory health care setting. They have the right to confidentiality. Even disclosing nonspecific information about AIDS may have consequences. A Texas high school received national news coverage when the number of HIV-positive cases was released. Discussion ensued about whether the statistics were accurate and whether the statistics should be revealed.

How do ambulatory heath care employees maximize the quality of remaining life for persons with AIDS and their families and significant others? If persons with AIDS are abandoned by family and friends and shunned at work, health care personnel may be their only human contact. A caring, compassionate attitude, which puts aside prejudices and value

TABLE 15-1
Health Care Workers with Documented and Possible Occupationally Acquired AIDS/HIV Infection, by Occupation, Reported through June 1997, United States[1]

Occupation	Documented occupational transmission[2] No.	Possible occupational transmission[3] No.
Dental worker, including dentist	—	7
Embalmer/morgue technician	—	2
Emergency medical technician/paramedic	—	10
Health aide/attendant	1	12
Housekeeper/maintenance worker	1	7
Laboratory technician, clinical	16	16
Laboratory technician, nonclinical	3	1
Nurse	21	29
Physician, nonsurgical	6	10
Physician, surgical	—	6
Respiratory therapist	1	2
Technician, dialysis	1	3
Technician, surgical	2	2
Technician/therapist, other than those listed above	—	5
Other health care occupations	—	2
Total	**52**	**114**

[1]Health care workers are defined as those persons, including students and trainess, who have worked in a health care, clinical, or HIV laboratory setting at any time since 1978. See *MMWR* 1992;41:823-25.

[2]Health care workers who had documented HIV seroconversion after occupational exposure or had other laboratory evidence of occupational infection: 45 had percutaneous exposure, 5 had mucocutaneous exposure, 1 had both percutaneous and mucocutaneous exposures, and 1 had an unknown route of exposure. Forty-seven exposures were to blood from an HIV-infected person, 1 to visibly bloody fluid, 1 to an unspecified fluid, and 3 to concentrated virus in a laboratory. Twenty-four of these health care workers developed AIDS.

[3]These health care workers have been investigated and are without indentifiable behavioral or transfusion risks; each reported percutaneous or mucocutaneous occupational exposures to blood or body fluids, or laboratory solutions containing HIV, but HIV seroconversion specifically resulting from an occupational exposure was not documented.

judgments, is to be fostered. Special care should be given to those individuals with organic brain damage who will need specific instructions and treatment information. Ambulatory health care employees must be informed about AIDS to prevent misinformation, rumor, apathy, and fear. Remember to care for the person and not the disease.

REFERENCES

1. Satcher, D: Centers for Disease Control and Prevention, HIV/AIDS Surveillance Report 8(1):3, 1996.
2. Ibid.
3. Ibid.
4. Burkett, E: How one nation Cuba stopped AIDS. The Seattle Times October 10, 1991.
5. AIDS and entrepreneurs. Hastings Cent Rep 20(6):3, 1991.

BIBLIOGRAPHY

Furrow, BR, et al: Health Law, Vol. 2. West, St Paul, Minn, 1995, pp 93–99, 196–207.
Galantino, ML: Clinical Assessment and Treatment of HIV. McGraw-Hill, New York, 1992.
Gentile, B: Doctors and AIDS. Newsweek July 1, 1991, p 48.
Gorman, C: The exorcist. Time 148(14):64, 1996.
Lindh, WQ, et al: Delmar's Comprehensive Medical Assisting Administrative and Clinical Competencies. Delmar, Albany, NY, 1998.
Marcil, WM, and Tigges, KN: The Person with AIDS. McGraw-Hill, New York, 1992.

Discussion Questions

1. *What are the advantages and disadvantages of mandatory testing for HIV?*

2. *If a child with AIDS were in your son's class at school, what do you think your community's response would be?*

3. *What precautions will you take if persons with AIDS are treated in the ambulatory health care setting where you are employed?*

4. *You have just learned cardiopulmonary resuscitation (CPR) and come upon an individual having a heart attack on the sidewalk. You have determined that CPR is necessary, but you also recall your class's discussion this morning of the transmission of AIDS. What will you do?*

5. *What would your reaction be if the spouse of one of your friends comes into the office for an AIDS blood test?*

6. *Check with your county health department to determine how AIDS is to be reported.*

16

Life and Death

Ted is 76 years old. He is retired and lives with his wife of 44 years and his adult daughter. As a laborer, he spent most of his working years with heavy equipment and cranes both on land and on tugs and ships, including salvage work. He loves the water. His home affords him the opportunity to look out on Puget Sound in the Pacific Northwest and watch the passing ships each day. Ted has been diagnosed with emphysema and suspected asbestosis. More than 7 years after diagnosis, his breathing is more difficult. His sense of humor, his love of life and his family, his care and concern for others, and his knowledge of the passing ships is as keen as ever.

LEARNING OBJECTIVES

Upon successful completion of this chapter, you will be able to:

1. Restate choices an individual might have in death.
2. Review at least three advances in technology that enhance or prolong life.
3. Define the term *euthanasia* and discuss its common usage.
4. Describe the living will, the advance directive, and durable power of attorney for health care.
5. Appraise components of the Patient Self-Determination Act.
6. Differentiate among various legal definitions of death.
7. Describe two famous court cases and their impact on prolonging life.
8. Express possible legal implications of life-and-death decisions.
9. Discuss at least three ethical implications of life-and-death decisions.
10. Define the role of the health professional in dealing with clients and families in life-and-death decisions.

DEFINITIONS

"Code Red." Medical slang indicating a life-or-death emergency.

Durable power of attorney for health care. Sometimes called medical proxy; the legal right to act on another's behalf in making health care decisions.

Euthanasia. From the Greek for "good death"; willfully causing or allowing death to keep a person with incurable disease from suffering; more commonly used today to express active euthanasia.

Living will. Legal document, voluntarily made by an adult, stating what treatment and procedures that person wants done in the event of a terminal illness, especially when the person is comatose or incompetent.

Patient Self-Determination Act. Federal law requiring institutions giving medical care to inform clients of their option to use advance directives such as living wills and durable powers of attorney for health care.

Physicians' directive. Washington State's response to the living will; sometimes called the Natural Death Act.

■ CHOICES IN LIFE AND DEATH

Throughout the text, many discussions of rights have surfaced both in the legal and in the bioethical sections. The right to health care, right to abortion, right to fertility choices, and right to privacy are just a few rights we claim for ourselves. In the last two decades, we have considered the alternatives in rights. Is health care a right or privilege? Is the right or privilege to a few or to everyone? Is the right to abortion ethical? Should fertility choices be available to all people and at what cost? How do we protect the right to confidentiality?

In dying, what choices do we have? How much of the choices in dying are personal decisions; how much is regulated or controlled by technology and advanced medicine?

Personal attitudes and public opinion have changed through the years. For example, in 1938 the Euthanasia Society of America was founded. It was a national, nonprofit organization dedicated to fostering communication about complex end-of-life decisions among individuals. The organization was best known for inventing the **living will** in 1967. In 1974 the Euthanasia Society was renamed Society for the Right to Die. In 1991 the Concern for Dying and the Society for the Right to Die merged to become Choice in Dying.

Public opinion that says we have a right to die and have choices in dying is indigenous to Western culture, which places so much emphasis on individual rights. Yet while we are increasingly seeking control over choices in dying, the power, the almost coercive power, of medical technology and medicine to preserve and prolong life will cause many of us to suffer years of debility, pain, and perhaps a lesser quality of life.

> Ted and his primary care internist are friends. They worship in the same church. When Ted sees his doctor, they tell each other jokes and swap stories. Then they get down to serious business and discuss his prognosis. Ted does not want to begin using oxygen. He sees that as the beginning of the end. He puts it off until he can no longer sleep peacefully. Even then, he uses oxygen only at night. Ted and his wife, Ann, discuss a living will; they talk with their daughter and son, who live away from home. Ted and Ann meet with the attorney, update their wills, and have the Washington State **physician's directive** executed. Ted shares it with his physician, and they agree on his care management.

Our desire to have choices in dying comes from fears and concerns related to prolonged dying as the result of technologic interventions. We would choose the refusal of treatment or hospitalization. Some might choose assisted suicide. Other individuals do not want to be a burden to significant others. They may fear becoming senile and dependent. Some may fear loss of control and want to choose their quality of life and have the choice of how they die. Medical technology offers insulin to control diabetes, a cardiac pacemaker or mechanical heart valves for a weak or diseased heart, renal dialysis for kidney failure, and angioplasty for clogged arteries.

> It is a cold and gloomy December. There is rain and even some snow in the Pacific Northwest. Ted is housebound most of the time now, but he still insists on driving Ann almost wherever she goes. His desire to get out, however, has lessened. The weather seems to make his breathing more labored. He is having serious headaches. It has been a few weeks since he has seen his doctor; however, when Ann suggests a visit, Ted grumbles that there is nothing more the doctor can do. One Sunday evening, Ted is unable to wear even his slippers because his feet and legs are so swollen. His humor is still active and he comments, "I feel like Jesus—walking on water." The water retention makes his feet feel like water pads. Ann decides to call the doctor the next morning.

Many who would be dead are alive because of technologic or mechanical intervention. Of the 2.2 million annual deaths in the United States, nearly 1.8 million will occur in health care facilities. And of those 1.8 million deaths, roughly 1.5 million were preceded by some deliberate decision to stop or not start medical treatment.[1]

Every day, medical personnel are confronted with more complex issues regarding the meaning of life and death. Where is the fine line between helping a person to live and allowing him or her to die? When is it appropriate to use extraordinary means to prolong life? What are extraordinary means? What are the legal implications if physicians withhold or withdraw treatment? Is there a difference between human need and human right? Who decides?

Each of us will die. From the moment we are born, we begin to die. Each day of life moves us closer to our death. Some of us will die suddenly and peacefully, perhaps in our sleep. Some of us will die suddenly as a result of an accident or as a victim of crime. Some of us will die slowly and gradually, with our bodies deteriorating and our organs ceasing to function. Some of us will die with little or no pain or discomfort. Some of us will die after great pain and discomfort. Most of us want to live, but when faced with death, we desire to go quickly, painlessly, and with dignity. However, not all of us will be so fortunate.

Consider the following example from Donald M. Hayes[2] in *Between Doctor and Patient:*

> *Mr. Baker had terminal kidney failure and was comatose. Several tubes came from various places in his body. He was receiving both blood and glucose into his veins. One night he went into cardiac arrest. A team of nurses and physicians responded with a "Code Red" and worked vigorously to resuscitate. The attempt was futile and Mr. Baker died. The memory of Mr. Baker's death was lasting to Mr. Rogers, the recently admitted patient in the same room. He said to his physician, "Please don't ever let that happen to me. I've tried all my life to live like a man; I want to die like one." Mr. Rogers underwent surgery that revealed inoperable, widespread cancer. He did not respond well, and a few days later he had a tube in his stomach, a catheter in his bladder, a tube through his nose, and intravenous tubes in both arms. When he suffered respiratory failure, a tracheotomy was performed to save his life. He was given a slate to write on, since a tracheotomy precludes speech. Later one evening, before he managed to switch off his respirator so that he might die peacefully, he wrote on the slate, "Doctor, remember; the enemy is not death. The enemy is inhumanity."*

Few for whom life has meaning would turn their backs on the medical technology that has added years of life for so many. Such advances in medicine are heralded by the public and the media; however, if not used judiciously, technology can supplant the quality of life. Technology has heightened our awareness of death at the same time that it increases our life span.

At some time in our lives, each of us will face the issue of how much medical technology to use to prolong life. Perhaps, too, we will wish for a "good death." Whether or not to prolong life may become a serious problem when the decision may be made with little forethought or adequate planning. When the physician tells a loved one that a cardiac pacemaker is necessary to regulate the heartbeat, the general response is, "When can it be done?"

The decision is more complex, however, when the loved one is hospitalized with a heart condition that is rapidly deteriorating and little can be done. The questions of how much intervention and when are much more serious. When the heart monitor indicates with a buzz and a continuous monotone sound that the heart has ceased to beat, somewhere, someone is going to ask, "Do we resuscitate?"

Early the next morning, Ted cannot breathe. He is suffocating. Ann dials 911. In minutes emergency medical technicians are at the door. In their quick assessment, they comment on how strong Ted's heart is but how weak his lungs are. Ann explains the emphysema and suspected asbestosis. After transportation to the hospital and treatment in the emergency room, Ted is moved to intensive care. Ann, their daughter, and their son are at his bedside. Although his breathing is now stabilized, the medical staff inquire about the use of a respirator. They indicate a willingness to abide by Ted's wishes but that it might be difficult if such action was necessary. They ask about a living will. The family responds positively. The Physician's Directive is later supplied to the hospital.

CHOICES IN DYING

Each of us wants to control his or her own life; especially we want power over dying. Maintaining that control may be easier envisioned and said than done. There may be many choices to make. We truly want a "good death" as much as we want a "good life." Given the ultimate power over choice, we would choose the good death, or **euthanasia.**

To use the term *euthanasia* in this context, however, is not so common today. Euthanasia has come to refer only to the active form, in which some action causes the death of another. This is in contrast to what might be called passive euthanasia, or the use of deliberate decisions that may result in death.

For example, are antibiotics prescribed when a hospitalized person contracts pneumonia and is suffering from the last stages of pancreatic cancer? Under what circumstances are "do not resuscitate" orders placed in clients' charts at hospitals or long-term care facilities?

Circumstances in the next few days greatly alter Ted's life. Ted's primary care physician and friend suffers his own tragedy. The physician's family is called to Denmark for a family death. When attempts to remove Ted's excess fluid are not totally successful, a nephrologist is called who advises that dialysis begin. The shunt is placed in Ted's shoulder, but neither Ted nor the family is anxious to begin dialysis. Ted had watched a close and dear friend suffer greatly, lose a limb, and eventually die after years of dialysis. Ted believes that dialysis will make it next to impossible for him to have a "good death." The nephrologist insists and discusses options with the substitute primary care physician. "This is just a 'jump start' to get your kidneys going; we will only have to dialyze you twice probably." Ted and Ann discuss the nephrologist's recommendations. There is hesitation, but the decision is finally made. When Ann is asked to sign the consent for dialysis, she comments to the hospital chaplain, who has been so attentive to the family, "Look at all these side effects." The chaplain explains the need to make individuals aware of all the possible side effects, but that few if any of them are likely to occur. Dialysis will begin the next morning.

Another person is being kept alive by a respirator. The client has no recognition and no awareness of surroundings. After careful assessment of the situation and a discussion and agreement with the family members, the medical staff turn off the equipment. Life support ceases. In a matter of minutes, the heart monitor indicates a flat line rather than a heartbeat. Death occurs.

How much pain medication will be prescribed for a client? If sufficient pain medication is prescribed to keep the terminally ill comfortable, health professionals understand that the very medication provided for pain relief also may depress breathing in some clients already so debilitated that the result may be to hasten death.

To ensure that we have choices in dying, there is legislation in all 50 states that allows us to make choices in death and to dictate to some extent to health care professionals our wishes.

LIVING WILLS, ADVANCE DIRECTIVES, AND THE PATIENT SELF-DETERMINATION ACT

Competent adults have always had the right to make choices about their health care, especially the right to forego life-sustaining treatments when death is imminent. Life-prolonging technology, however, advanced further and faster than did health care professionals. Incompetent adults also needed to voice their choices in dying.

More and more often, health care professionals, especially physicians, found themselves in legal and ethical dilemmas with little or no direction from the legal community. Across the country, states began to pass legislation that gave clients the legal right to forego life-sustaining treatments, nutrition, and hydration and provided protection to physicians and hospitals carrying out such orders. Such directives allow individuals or their representatives to make decisions regarding their dying.

California and Washington were forerunners in such legislation. California's document was the **living will;** Washington's response to the legal dilemma was the **physicians' directive,** or Natural Death Act. In addition, the federal government passed the **Patient Self-Determination Act,** sponsored by Senators John C. Danforth (R.-Missouri) and Daniel Patrick Moynihan (D.-New York), which became effective December 1, 1991.

This law applies to all health care institutions receiving payments from medicare and medicaid. These institutions include hospitals, skilled nursing facilities, hospices, home care programs, and health maintenance organizations. Physicians become involved when their practice interacts with these institutions. The Patient Self-Determination Act requires that all adult persons who receive medical care from such institutions be given written information about their right to accept or refuse medical or surgical treatment. These clients must also be given information about their right to formulate advance directives such as living wills and to designate someone to act on their behalf in making health care decisions (**durable power of attorney for health care,** or medical proxy) (see Appendix II).[3]

Ann and her son and daughter return to their homes for a good night's rest before their return to the hospital early the next morning. The weather, however, intervens. Heavy snow fell during the night. The hills of Seattle are clogged with vehicles going nowhere. Freeways are treacherous. Even the streets to the hospital are impassable. Dialysis technicians and portable dialysis machines are delayed. Their load backs up and patients more critical than Ted wait long past their dialysis time for treatment. Ted's condition worsens. Fortunately, the weather moderates, and dialysis begins. It does little to help, however. More than two treatments pass. Ted begins to bleed internally, and his laboratory tests indicate that an emergency exists. The substitute physician has now left for his Christmas vacation. A surgeon is called in—another stranger to the family, but the "freshest" one available. It seems every surgeon and every hospital is overburdened this Christmas holiday. Emergency surgery is scheduled

> for 5 PM. The family is at the bedside. But there is to be another delay. The operating room is full; a code red in the room Ted is to use delays Ted's surgery. Ted's condition becomes so critical that the surgeon checks with other nearby hospitals for an available operating room. None is available. Finally, at 1 AM Ted is taken to the operating room. By now the family has been told that there is only a 50–50 chance he will survive.

The actual implementation of the Patient Self-Determination Act remained a matter for the states. In 1992, Pennsylvania became the 50th state to enact advance directive legislation. The Patient Self-Determination Act, however, does not override any state law allowing a health care provider to object on the basis of conscience in the implementation of such an advance directive.

▬▬ DURABLE POWER OF ATTORNEY FOR HEALTH CARE

In addition to living wills or physicians' directives, many individuals choose to use the durable power of attorney or the **durable power of attorney for health care,** legal documents that add another dimension to the decision-making process. Although the living will or physicians' directive allows the writer to determine whether heroic or extraordinary measures will be used, the durable power of attorney allows an agent to act on an individual's behalf in additional ways.

The durable power of attorney is a legal form that allows a designated person to act on another's behalf. Likewise, the durable power of attorney for health care or the medical proxy more specifically allows a designated person to make only health care decisions for another. This proxy or person becomes an agent, or attorney-in-fact. This agent may be a spouse, a grown child, a close friend, or other relative or someone in whom the person has full confidence. A person must be competent to sign a power of attorney. Some states require that the signer must be able to manage his or her own property effectively at the time of signing. The reason for signing a power of attorney is to ensure that someone will be around to act for a person who becomes physically or mentally disabled. The signer keeps control over the signed legal form as long as the person can manage independently. The signed document can be given to a lawyer or a close friend with instructions that it should not be turned over to the attorney-in-fact unless the need arises. Once signed, the document is in effect until it is revoked.

The designated person who acts on behalf of the client should know and understand the client's living will. What would happen if the power of attorney acted in violation of the client's living will? No court has taken action to see who would prevail. Thus it is wise to ensure that the power of attorney will act on the client's behalf in all instances of health care.

Ted's surgery lasts 4 hours. Ted survives; but he is returned to the intensive care unit (ICU) on a respirator. There has been a bowel perforation and one-half of his colon has been removed. He remains critical, but amazingly is able to be weaned from his respirator in 24 hours. By now Ted is receiving food and hydration, blood, platelets, antibiotics, and pain medication intravenously. He cannot speak, but is somewhat alert. He is seriously weakened. Urine output decreases and the question of dialysis returns. At this point, all persons involved in Ted's care meet to discuss treatment. The decision is made to meet with the family. Ann and her daughter and son are interviewed separately about their wishes and Ted's wishes regarding extraordinary means. Earlier an ICU nurse had told the family that if even one of them has any hesitation about treatment, the hospital would not be able to follow Ted's wishes. After completion of the interviews, it is clear that the family intends to follow Ted's wishes. Dialysis would cease. It is only a matter of time now. The nephrologist, however, has other ideas. When she discovers dialysis has discontinued, she demands to know why. When the family explains, she says, "I was not present for that consultation. I will have to hear it from Ted myself." She goes to Ted's bedside, asks him if he can understand her, and says, "Ted, do you want dialysis?" Ted, in his hospital bed with head and shoulders elevated 10 to 20 degrees, has his arms immobilized at his side for the drip of numerous IV lines. An oxygen mask covers his nose and mouth. His eyes show lack of rest and sleep, fear for what is happening to him, and concern for his family. Ted shrugs his shoulders and opens his hands palms upward in gesture. The nephrologist is ordering a chest x-ray and dialysis when the family intervenes. An on-call physician and the nephrologist argue outside Ted's room, in earshot of the family. The attending physician indicates that in Ted's condition, dialysis probably will do more harm than good. His body cannot withstand dialysis. But the nephrologist is determined.

Each state has established rules governing the use of the durable power of attorney. Professional legal advice regarding a given state's stipulations and requirements may be advisable, but preprinted forms are available in most stationery stores. See Appendix II for an example of a durable power of attorney for health care used in Washington.

When there seems no hope and the family is feeling powerless, their family physician returns from Denmark. Dialysis treatment ceases again, but the damage has already been done. Ted has suffered not just one but all of the possible side effects that Ann has read about. Ted is bleeding internally now from almost every organ of his body. All IVs are removed except what is needed to remain to keep Ted comfortable. Every breath is the hardest work his body has ever known. Each member of the family, in his or her own way, says good-bye and tells Ted how much he is loved. Nurses and doctors who have been so attentive in the previous 25 days also stop by. The ICU nurses continue to do what they are best known for—attending to the needs of the critically ill. The primary care physician remains close. The end is peaceful. The end is relief. Relief from agony and pain. Relief from any more difficult decisions. Relief from the disappointment that a loved one's wishes could be so hard to carry out.

LEGAL DEFINITIONS OF DEATH

An early legal definition of death was the cessation of the heart and lung wherein the two were so interrelated that the cessation of one leads to the cessation of another, followed by the cessation of all cognitive activity, all other brain functions, and all responsiveness in general. The cessation of the heart and of breathing was the simplest to identify and the easiest test of life, and it became the acceptable definition of death. Today the vast majority of deaths in the United States are determined by this traditional definition of death.[4]

With medical technologic advances, resuscitative devices, increased complexities of life, and organ transplants, the heart-lung definition of death was found insufficient. Death is a continuum, and different parts of the body die at different times. The heart may stop before or after the client dies. For example, in a heart attack victim, the heart stops beating, but the client does not die immediately. Approximately 3 to 4 minutes pass before there is irreparable brain death. At this point, the client is dead. Once the brain dies, there is no need for the other body organs, and they die at various intervals.[5]

Subsequently, the concept of brain death was presented by the Harvard Ad-Hoc Committee, chaired by Henry Beecher. The criteria were simple: A client in this state appears to be in deep coma. The condition can be satisfactorily diagnosed by the following points: (1) unreceptivity and unresponsitivity, (2) no movements or breathing, (3) no reflexes, and (4) a flat electroencephalogram. Each of these tests shall be repeated at least 24 hours later with no change.[6] This definition of brain death does not cover cases such as Karen Ann Quinlan, who was in a persistent vegetative state, or people who are in comas but do not meet other accepted criteria.

In 1983 President Ronald Reagan formed a commission to discuss the ethical implications of dying and death. The commission's report, entitled "Deciding to Forego Life-Sustaining Treatment," recommended that all U.S. jurisdictions accept the Uniform Determination of Death Act. The act was developed under the commission's direction by three organizations: the American Bar Association, the American Medical Association, and the National Conference of Commissioners on Uniform State Laws. The act "established that the irreversible cessation of all circulatory and respiratory functions, or irreversible cessation of all functions of the entire brain, including the brain stem" is the criterion of death.[7] The commission further stated that such a definition ought to incorporate general physiologic standards rather than medical criteria or tests that would change with advances in medical technology.

Some believed that the higher brain death definition addresses all purposes. This definition is the permanent and irreversible cessation of all higher brain or neocortical functions. There is no medical test to determine higher brain function; therefore it is doubtful that this definition will become a legally acceptable one. The higher brain death definition may allow a greater allowance of who is "dead," and would allow those with cognitive impairments to be "buried."

Last, there are some who believe that individuals should be allowed to choose their own personal definition of death and one that fits their own values and interests. Of course, there is no medical test to determine these. This definition is not legally acceptable.

Whatever the state's legal definition of death, the declaration of death will be made by medical standards as are defined in the Uniform Determination of Death Act. This means that as technology changes and medicine advances, laws will not necessarily change; rather, good medical practices will determine what counts as good evidence that the legal definition of death has occurred. With the heart-lung definition, there may be some leeway on the part of the physician to determine death. For example, if a relative is traveling to the dying client, the physician may choose to keep the client alive until the relative says good-bye. Further, when a physician declares a person dead, that physician should not be involved in the transplantation of organs, although this is not required by law. Transplantation is discussed in Chapter 17.

◼️ LEGAL IMPLICATIONS

Most legal rulings on life and death center around "Who decides?" Prolonging life by artificial means usually poses few legal problems. Federal laws state that kidney clients have the right to funding and the use of kidney dialysis machines. Some means of prolonging life artificially, such as insulin administration, are so easy, inexpensive, and widely practiced that there is no controversy about their use. On the other hand, some procedures, such as dialysis, are so expensive that federal legislation was necessary to ensure that every citizen has the right to such treatments regardless of cost.

Choices in dying, however, are complex and controversial. Consider case law in the following two circumstances. In seeking greater choice in the process of dying, the courts appear to be regulating in a more restrictive manner. Is litigation the driving force behind health care professionals and the institutions they serve not wanting to abide by clients' known choices in dying? Is there a general feeling that we do indeed have rights, but the right to die or to make our own choices about dying is not so carefully protected?

The litigation over the case of Karen Ann Quinlan was widely publicized. Quinlan was a New Jersey woman who, at age 21, was taken to the hospital in a comatose state by friends after a birthday party. No one is sure exactly what happened to Karen on Tuesday, April 14, 1975, but the world soon began to follow her life closely. Her case was a newsworthy first. Karen's condition deteriorated. On July 31, her parents gave her physicians permission to take Karen off the respirator and signed a letter to that effect. The physicians disagreed with the decision on moral grounds and refused to take Karen off the respirator. Legal action ensued. On September 12 the attorney for Joseph Quinlan, Karen's father, filed a plea with the Superior Court on three constitutional grounds: (1) the right to privacy, (2) religious freedom, and (3) cruel and unusual punishment.

Judge Rober Muir ruled against Joseph Quinlan, who then appealed the decision to the New Jersey Supreme Court. The court's decision was in Joseph Quinlan's favor and set aside any criminal liability for removing the respirator. It further recommended that Karen's physicians consult the hospital ethics committee to concur with their prognosis for Karen. Weeks later Karen was weaned from the machine.[8] She lived until 1986.

In the nearly 20 years since the Quinlan case, similar cases have caused emotional trauma to families faced with the death of a loved one. Many such cases have been publicized in the media. In 1983 Nancy Cruzan was in an auto accident, sustained severe injuries, was declared incompetent, and was referred to as being in a persistent vegetative state. The physicians treated her aggressively, but she remained in a coma for 3 weeks before she was able to take any nutrition by mouth. Eventually, a gastrostomy and hydration tube was placed directly into her stomach for ease in feeding and comfort. The state of Missouri bore the cost of her care.

In 1989 Nancy's parents, aware of their daughter's wishes, requested that the hospital terminate her artificial nutrition and hydration and allow her to die. It was known that Nancy had virtually no chance of recovering her cognitive abilities. The state hospital refused. Nancy's parents then took legal action. The state trial court authorized the termination, finding that a person in Cruzan's condition has a fundamental right under the Missouri Constitution and the U.S. Constitution to direct or refuse the withdrawal of life-prolonging procedures.

The State Supreme Court reversed in 1990, and later the U.S. Supreme Court affirmed the decision of the State Supreme Court. The U.S. Supreme Court stated that there was no clear and convincing evidence of Nancy's desire to have hydration and nutrition withdrawn under such circumstances. The fact that Nancy's previous roommate could recall conversations that Nancy did not want to live as a "vegetable," and other observations to the same effect, was not enough to convince the court. The observations did not deal in terms of withdrawal of medical treatment or of hydration and nutrition. The U.S. Supreme Court, however, recognized that the right to refuse medical treatment is guaranteed by the U.S. Constitution rather than in case law. Nancy Cruzan died in December 1990.

Both Quinlan and Cruzan were alive when their cases were brought before the courts. The question in both cases was whether each woman should be kept alive, one by use of a respirator, the other by receiving artificial hydration and nutrition. It was not whether they were legally dead. Their parents both were asking "Should they be allowed to die?" What do you think? What impact should medical technology have on these decisions? Who pays? Who should decide? Is it more difficult to remove hydration and nutrition than a respirator?

■ ETHICAL CONSIDERATIONS

Life-and-death choices are numerous. The many factors to consider include the following: Who makes the decision? Whose right is paramount—the client's or the health care provider's? Do circumstances influence decisions? If so, what are they? What is ordinary and extraordinary treatment? Should resuscitation be started? Should treatment be withheld?

Who makes the decision is not easy to determine. Clients like to believe they do. Many times physicians alone decide. The government, through state statutes, may determine who shall live or die. The burden of such decisions is heavy. If a decision is required in an emergency life-and-death matter, those in closest proximity to the client will decide.

In health care facilities, the law may determine who decides. A main function of such facilities is to preserve life. If there is any question, consideration is given to the wishes of the client, the wishes of the family, the recommendations of the physician, and perhaps the recommendations of a professional team of individuals whose purpose it is to make a decision.

The problem arises over whose right is paramount in a decision. At times it is obvious. If a client is unable to decide, for whatever reason, others have to be involved. The family has an influence. The cases of Karen Ann Quinlan and Nancy Cruzan demonstrated that the influence of family is not decisive, however. The same often is true of a client's wishes. Even if clients are able to express their wishes to physicians and health care providers, circumstances may override them. Consider, for example, an elderly client with a physicians' directive who communicates that he wishes to die at home. He nears death and has difficulty breathing. His family members call emergency help. Paramedics, of necessity and training, use heroic measures to prevent death and then transport the client to the nearest hospital. In this case, it is best for family members to recognize that such actions may circumvent the client's choice and the physicians' directive.

Many circumstances influence decisions. Age is a factor. Resuscitation may be started on a 16-year-old and not on an 89-year-old. Cost is also a factor. Triple cardiac bypass surgery may be performed for someone of substantial means more readily than for the indigent derelict. Health is a factor. A pacemaker may be inserted for the elderly client whose general health is good, but it may not be used if the client's health is poor and other severe physical difficulties exist. The availability of resources is a factor. With only one kidney and four needy persons, three will do without.

Other factors may be religion, personal philosophy of life, the amount of pain one can endure, whether a client is comatose, and what the client's feelings are on a good life versus a good death. All these factors are relative. Some are old at age 45; others are young at 90. Some can endure great pain, and others have a low threshold for pain. What is poor health to one person may seem to be good health to another. The relativity of the factors complicates the decision and mandates that each decision be considered individually on its own merits.

No one ethical guideline is adequate for a statement on choices in dying. One ethical view is that euthanasia is murder because of either omission or commission. Tied closely with this view are the thoughts that only God has the right to decide at what moment a person should die and that euthanasia violates the biblical command "Thou shalt not kill." Some religious groups believe suffering is part of the divine plan for every person.

A careful examination of these attitudes prompts such thoughts as, "God wants each of us to live, but when it comes time to die, cannot possibly wish a bad death for anyone." Often the proponents of "Thou shalt not kill" have no difficulty with killing on the battlefield and will go to great lengths to justify war biblically.

The possibility also exists that clients pronounced incurable may recover, which would be impossible if euthanasia already had been committed. Clients suffering greatly may request to die on the spur of the moment with little thought of the ramifications.

Some people believe that legal euthanasia or physician-assisted suicide would weaken the moral fiber of the country and may lead to such actions for eugenic reasons. If we can bring death for one individual to prevent further suffering, why not for severely deformed infants who have no possibility of a "normal" life? Consider the circumstances of an infant born with severe congenital defects and intestinal obstructions requiring surgery. The medical staff and parents may decide not to operate and let the infant die. Allowing this to occur is not easy. It means watching a tiny infant gradually dehydrate and suffer from infection for a period of perhaps days. The ordeal can be terrible. Parents are protected from this experience, but the medical staff is not. Many physicians and health professionals ask, "Would it not be more merciful to inject the infant with a lethal dose of medication that would cause death to come quickly and painlessly and prevent the suffering?"

Perhaps even more personal and difficult questions are, How do I want to die? What kind of lifesaving measures would I want? Do I prefer active euthanasia or physician-assisted suicide? Can I stand to suffer? Do I have any control over my own death? Do I have a right to die as I choose? What would I want health professionals to do for me?

■■■ THE ROLE OF HEALTH PROFESSIONALS IN AMBULATORY CARE

Ambulatory health care employees will make life-and-death decisions only in personal relationships with their families and friends, rather than in any professional capacity. They often may, however, be involved in conversations with clients or their families who are struggling with the question. They also may be sounding boards to physicians involved in the decision-making process.

Ambulatory health care employees do not make death decisions in any professional capacity. Their physician employers, however, do. Certainly the law should be followed, religious practices considered, and the client's rights protected when possible, but no clearly established guideline is available.

Clients who willingly and openly discuss their beliefs and wishes concerning their own deaths should be encouraged to complete living wills or physicians' directives. Legal counsel should be recommended to people if appropriate. Clients should not be made to feel ashamed or guilty because of their feelings about death, no matter how much they differ from yours.

Ambulatory care employees and physicians must be understanding and compassionate. Every attempt must be made to respect the feelings of clients and their families. Families should be allowed to express any guilt they may feel in making decisions. A clear picture of the circumstances, explained by the physician in words clients can comprehend, can alleviate much of that problem. Clients who have strong feelings about having their lives prolonged should be encouraged to make their wishes known.

When physicians or employees are confronted with situations or questions they cannot handle, consultations and referrals should be sought. Attorneys may be called, and medical societies may offer assistance. Hospital ethics committees may be valuable. Hospital chaplains, staff psychiatrists, and social workers are specially trained to help others with these personal and professional issues. Decisions of the kind discussed in this chapter weigh heavily on the minds of those involved. That weight should not be allowed to become too great.

REFERENCES

1. Kass, LR: Is there a right to die? Hastings Cent Rep 25(1):34, 1993.
2. Hayes, DM: Between Doctor and Patient. Judson Press, Valley Forge, Pa, 1977, pp 9–11.
3. Preparing for Advance Directives, Thursday, June 27, 1991. American Hospital Association, pp 8–11.
4. Furrow, BR et al: Health Law, Vol 2. West, St Paul, Minn, 1995, pp 306–307.
5. Barnard, C: Good Life. Good Death. Prentice-Hall, Englewood Cliffs, NJ, 1980, pp 6–7.
6. Yezzi, R: Medical Ethics. Holt, Rinehart & Winston, New York, 1980, p 113.
7. Annas, GJ, Glantz, LH, and Katz, BF: The Rights of Doctors, Nurses and Allied Health Professionals. Avon Books, New York, 1981, p 228.
8. Munson, R: Intervention and Reflection: Basic Issues in Medical Ethics. Wadsworth, Belmont, Calif, 1992, p 147.

BIBLIOGRAPHY

Ames, K: Last rights. Newsweek August 26, 1991, pp 40–41.
Annas, GJ: Nancy Cruzan in China. Hastings Cent Rep 20(5):39, 1990.
Begley, S: Choosing death. Newsweek August 26, 1991, pp 40–46.
Capron, AM: Baby Ryan and virtual futility. Hastings Cent Rep 25(2):20, 1995.
Capron, AM: Constitutionalizing death. Hastings Cent Rep 25(12):23, 1995.
Capron, AM: Even in defeat, Proposition 161 sounds a warning. Hastings Cent Rep 23(1):32, 1993.
Capron, AM: Sledding in Oregon. Hastings Cent Rep 25(1):34, 1995.
Dying Well? A Colloquy on Euthanasia and Assisted Suicide. Hastings Cent Rep 22(2), 1992. (A series of nine euthanasia and assisted suicide articles by different authors.)
Gibbs, N: Love and let die. Time March 19, 1990, pp 62–71.
Hendin, H: Selling death and dignity. Hastings Cent Rep 25(3):19, 1995.
Hill, TP: Pa. and N.J. differ on the right to die. The Philadelphia Inquirer May 15, 1992.

Lippman, H: Legally speaking after Cruzan: The right to die. RN January:65.

Lyle, KL: A gentle way to die. Newsweek March 2, 1992, p 14.

Morreim, EH: Profoundly diminished life: The casualties of coercion. Hastings Cent Rep 24(1):33, 1994.

Schneider, CE: Making sausage: The ninth circuit's opinion. Hastings Cent Rep 27(1):27, 1997.

Truog, RD: Is it time to abandon brain death? Hastings Cent Rep 27(1):29, 1997.

Veatch, RM: The impending collapse of the whole-brain definition of death. Hastings Cent Rep 23(4):18, 1993.

Wilson, V: Old, sick and far away. Newsweek August 26, 1991, p 39.

Wolf, SM: Final exit: The end of argument. Hastings Cent Rep 21(1):30, 1992.

Discussion Questions

1. *Refer to the example of Baker and Rogers at the beginning of the chapter. What would you do if you were the physician? What would you do if you were a loved one? Would your actions cause any difficulties? If so, describe.*

2. *If you knew you would be put in the same situation as Karen Ann Quinlan or Nancy Cruzan, what would you wish? Why?*

3. *Describe the circumstances in which a client might be unable to make a decision on prolonging life.*

4. *A family member comes to the ambulatory health care setting. She is angry because the hospital "won't stop their endless testing" and "keeps trying the impossible with my husband." What is your response?*

5. *A surgical client with a guarded prognosis initiates a conversation with the physician: "If I'm not going to make it, don't let me suffer." How can the physician respond?*

6. *Under what circumstances might physicians and family members choose not to initiate heroic measures for a client?*

7. *How would you deal with the situation if you were a nurse in a hospital nursery in which orders from the medical staff and family indicate "do not feed" for a genetically deformed infant?*

8. *How would you deal with the husband who opted for euthanasia as requested by his wife? The spouse is not sure he has made the right decision, and his adult children are critical of his decision.*

9. *In the case of Ted, in which conflict arose among Ted, the family, and the medical professionals, where ultimately does the power reside? Explain your answer. Discuss your personal reaction to Ted's case. What went right and what went wrong?*

17 *Dying and Death*

LEARNING OBJECTIVES

Upon successful completion of this chapter, you will be able to:

1. List at least eight generalizations about suffering and dying.
2. Compare short- and long-term suffering.
3. Describe the importance of medications for dying clients.
4. Identify and explain at least five psychologic factors affecting dying clients.
5. Identify and explain at least five physiologic factors affecting dying clients.
6. Discuss the stages of dying as defined by Kubler-Ross.
7. Describe the services of hospices for dying clients.
8. Differentiate between active euthanasia and physician-assisted suicide.
9. Discuss the Uniform Anatomical Gift Act.
10. Describe an autopsy and who may authorize one.
11. Explain the role of physicians and ambulatory health care employees in dying and death.

Death is the final stage of life. Dying is a process or a preparation for the final conclusion—death. For some, *dead* is a four-letter word not to be discussed; to others, the word represents an unpleasant reality difficult to think about or plan for. Some handle the concept realistically and well. In many respects, the way people face their dying or their death may be determined by how they live.

Most health care professionals will work with clients who die and will respond to their surviving loved ones. How health professionals face this process may also be determined, in part, by how they face their own life and their own death. With the added knowledge of this chapter on dying and death, health care professionals will be better prepared to work with clients and their families during the dying-and-death process. Caring, understanding, and compassion are essential ingredients.

▐▬▬ SUFFERING IN DYING

Dying and suffering are personal events. No two people suffer and die alike. To attempt to identify any particular models in suffering and dying is fruitless. None exists. Each person is unique, and the life experiences brought to the situation are varied. However, some generalizations can be made.

1. The way people live is often mirrored in the way they die.
2. People with useful support systems, such as friends, family, and faith in life, may find this support helpful in dying.
3. Experiencing the death of someone close brings the reality of dying into focus.
4. Intellectual preparation for dying, such as writing a will and an obituary or planning a funeral, may ease the fear of death.
5. Relationships with families and friends change.
6. Basic personalities usually remain unchanged, but moods may vary radically.
7. Personal goals are reevaluated.
8. Pain, suffering, and dependence are feared most by the dying.
9. Dying is not a casual experience.
10. The age of dying persons in part determines their reaction to death.
11. Cultural mores influence attitudes toward death.

Short-term suffering presents a set of problems different from those of long-term suffering. This can best be seen in the following situations:

Example 1
A 45-year-old teacher learned in June that chronic myelocytic leukemia accompanied by blastic transformation was destroying his body. The prognosis was poor. Hospitalization and chemotherapy followed, with severe side effects and pain. He died 2 months later, never returning home.

Example 2

A 50-year-old electrician was diagnosed as having cancer of the colon. Surgery followed, and a permanent colostomy was established. Postoperatively, the client did well and later returned to work part-time. Within a year, cancer metastasized and complications resulted. Consultation with specialists recommended only symptomatic treatment. Her pain required massive doses of analgesics to keep her comfortable for the remaining 6 months. The electrician was unable to return to work but remained home until about 6 weeks before death, when she was again hospitalized.

In a comparison of these two illustrations, time, costs, and dependency are three variables to consider. Obviously, the time of pain and suffering is longer for the electrician than for the teacher. The severity, however, cannot be compared. Overall costs are far greater for the electrician than the teacher, but nothing is known of insurance coverage or family resources. Either situation could be a financial burden on survivors. Dependency of these clients on their friends and family is somewhat different. The teacher had to depend on someone to take care of any personal matters, which might include job, children, and finances, for approximately 2 months. The electrician, however, was dependent on family for physical and nursing care in the home. She also needed someone to take care of personal matters from diagnosis to death, approximately 18 months.

Even the length of time is difficult to establish. Time is relative; that is, 2 months and 18 months may both be considered short-term when compared with an individual in a state of semiconsciousness for 4 or 5 years.

USE OF MEDICATIONS

Medications are used by the suffering when dying both in the hospital and at home. The greatest difficulty with medications arises in long-term suffering.

Medications are given for many reasons, including analgesics for pain, sedatives for sleep, and specific medications for the particular disease condition. Antidepressants and tranquilizers also may be prescribed. Medications are to be respected for their intended action and the client's needs.

Problems arise when family members, friends, and even allied health professionals circumvent or question the physician's orders for medications. This is often disastrous for the client. All persons close to the client ought to understand the physician's orders and the use of the prescribed medications. Family members should know the reasoning of the physician so that any questions arising are not misunderstood. For example, imagine the fear a loved one feels when the pharmacist says, "Do you know this is a near-lethal dose?" Unless the loved one knows that this amount is needed to keep the pain level of the client bearable, the loved one may withhold the medication and even begin to distrust the physician. Family members need to understand that medications may be given in different dosages, frequencies, and combinations for a dying client than for others. Age, weight, illness (whether chronic or acute), and the client's threshold for pain all influence a physician's choice of analgesics.

Sometimes physicians and health care professionals are reluctant to prescribe or administer medications even though it is an approved dosage range. In fact, in some cases health care professionals will administer less than the prescribed dose because they believe what was prescribed was too much. Some may fear the client will become addicted. Physicians may see narcotic orders or prescriptions as crimes, not as treatment issues. They fear investigation. The client or family may want less than prescribed because they believe it is too much. Clients may wait too long to ask for pain medication, thinking they "can handle it." All have the potential of working against the clients' comfort.

■■■ PSYCHOLOGIC ASPECTS OF DYING

Dying clients differ in their psychologic experiences. Although basic personalities remain the same, changes occur. A person normally calm and loving may have periods of violence and hostility. A happy person may become severely depressed. In fact, a person who is nearly comatose or close to death may be unaware of their responses to questions or be unable to make any decisions. An individual who usually is able to accept medical fact may totally deny a life-threatening illness.

Relationships may change. Some individuals are incapable of continuing a close relationship with a person who is dying. Closest friends may become aloof and distant. Some may fear touching or caressing the dying person. The dying person may reject any close contact or relationships. The following quotation, words from a dying person, illustrates this controversy. "I am not sure why, but I want to accept, and end up rejecting; I am willing to surrender, but more often seek to control."[1] The opposite may also be true. A stronger bond of friendship can develop, and new friendships will be made, possibly from individuals in similar circumstances. Broken relationships may be healed.

Relationships are important and should be encouraged. They provide strength and support that may not be available through any other source. The depth of relationships during this time and the degree of acceptance by dying clients may depend on their self-image. When a person is ill, is in pain, lives in a deteriorating body, and possibly is unable to perform the activities of daily living, self-image is fragile. When self-image is lacking, hope is lost; dying clients feel useless, may think they are burdens, and will have difficulties accepting help. The psychologic effect of a poor self-image may even hasten death.

Dying clients may not be physically able to continue working. If they are sole wage earners, this may present a financial crisis, especially if the unemployed period extends for a long time. Unemployed clients may be bored, feel useless, and worry, and their self-image suffers. For example, dying clients may worry that they are not fulfilling their usual role in the family and worry about their lack of control.

Personal goals for the dying person are altered or may even become nonexistent. Goals such as seeing a child graduate or a grandchild born may be seen as unrealistic to the dying because of limited time. The dying either give up or strive to live to that event. The total loss of personal goals, no matter how insignificant they may appear, can be devastating to the dying and to persons caring for them. Indecision is often a psychologic dilemma accompanying the lack of personal goals. People close to the dying commonly recommend goals and help in the decision-making process. This must be done sensitively and realistically.

Communication may become difficult. Aside from any psychologic problems, what dying clients are unable to understand or hear may depend on what they choose to hear or are ready to understand. Communication may be complicated further if the client's condition has not been honestly addressed. Of course, the opposite may be true. Some dying clients express the ability to communicate with greater depth because of the urgency of their circumstances.

Many communication difficulties center around the question of whether dying clients should be told of their terminal condition. How much information should they be given? Some people believe that all clients need to be told the medical facts by physicians and treated openly and honestly by all health professionals. They believe informed clients are better able to face death and are less afraid of the truth than are many health professionals. Other people believe no clients should be told they are dying, or that only those clients who give some verbal or nonverbal indication that they want to know should be told. Only clients who can handle the truth should be told. Some clients may refuse to set goals, give up hope, and wait impatiently for death.

Fear is often a traumatic psychologic aspect of dying. There is fear of pain, fear of long suffering, fear of losing independence, fear of financial ruin, and fear of death itself. The client's fears ought to be recognized and alleviated, if possible. To recognize these fears requires active and passive listening on the part of all people close to the dying individual and a willingness on the part of this individual to express those fears.

Much fear can be lessened if people close to the dying anticipate the fear and provide possible solutions and appropriate resources. Outside help may be sought, if necessary. Social workers, public health nurses, home health aides, clergy, and other health professionals can be valuable resources. Clients' fear should be taken seriously, and reference to their unimportance should be avoided.

The psychologic aspects of death are difficult for family, physicians, and ambulatory health care personnel because they may not be tangible. They generally are less understood than the physiologic aspects of death and are often left to laypersons rather than professionals. To care for the physical and ignore the psychologic is to treat only half the client.

■■■■ PHYSIOLOGIC ASPECTS OF DYING

Medicine has numerous treatments for some of the physiologic problems of suffering and pain experienced in the dying process. Sometimes the treatments are sufficient; other times, they barely address the problem. Untreated or undiagnosed physiologic problems may cause or enhance psychologic difficulties for dying clients.

Separating the psychologic from the physiologic is difficult. For example, pain and suffering, if untreated by therapy or medicinal means, may prove to be a psychologic barrier for clients, their families, and health professionals.

Loss of communication skills, such as in the aphasic client or in the comatose client, may be frustrating and unbearable. If clients are indecisive or senile because of physiologic changes, they may not be able to participate in the decision-making process of their terminal illness. Family members may need to assume greater roles in talking for clients and making decisions.

Other common physiologic problems encountered include loss of bodily functions; inability to move or ambulate; inability to eat or drink; and inability to tolerate medications, treatments, light, or sound. In the hospital setting, these symptoms may be treated without much difficulty. However, if clients choose to die at home, professional help or training may prove valuable. If clients become severely handicapped physically, they may be reluctant to go anywhere, even to the ambulatory health care setting. Family members may become exhausted caring for them or be unable to administer some of their treatments. The more severe these physiologic problems, the more difficult daily existence becomes.

Physiologic difficulties may hinder sexual identity and involvement. Dying clients' sexuality may be affected. It may be difficult or impossible to participate in sexual intercourse. The physiologic and psychologic aspects of sexuality are so intertwined that cause and effect are difficult to determine. A discussion of sexuality and related client problems needs to be initiated with the client and partner.

Physiologic and psychologic problems are to be anticipated, diagnosed, and treated. Treating the physiologic and psychologic aspects of clients enables total client care.

STAGES OF GRIEF

Elisabeth Kubler-Ross defines five stages or responses of dying: denial, anger, bargaining, depression, and acceptance. There is no set period for any one stage, nor will every dying person go through every stage. Some may stay in denial until death; others may manage denial and bargaining and stumble in depression. Still others may move back and forth from one stage to another. Some may move through some or all of the stages several times. There is no set or acceptable pattern. Each dying client is an individual, as are family members. However, the stages do offer information on how to relate to clients and their families, who will experience similar stages.

Elisabeth Kubler-Ross defines five stages of dying:
1. Denial
2. Anger
3. Bargaining
4. Depression
5. Acceptance

Denial

Clients may deny their terminal illness or go through periods of disbelief. Sometimes it is a result of shock when they are first told. Clients commonly say, "This is not happening to me" or "I'll go to another physician to see what's wrong." Denial generally is a temporary defense and offers therapeutic meaning to clients. Medical health care employees want to listen to clients during this stage. Trying to contradict clients or force them to believe what is happening to them will be to no avail. Encourage clients to talk about death. Listen, listen, listen.

Anger

Clients suddenly realize, "It is me. This is happening to me. Why me?" They may become "problem clients" and are envious and resentful. Anger may be dispersed in all directions, at people and toward the environment. Rage and temper tantrums can occur. Professionals and family members need to be understanding no matter how angry the client becomes. Listening to clients is important to allow them to vent their own feelings.

Bargaining

During this stage, clients try to make deals with physicians, God, or family, usually for more time or for a period of comfort without pain. Clients tend to be more cooperative and congenial. Common responses include the following: "Please let me see my homeland again." "I'll be so good, if I can just have 3 pain-free hours." "Dear God, I'll never . . . if you make me well." Medical health care employees can listen to dying clients' requests but not become a party to the bargain. Some bargaining may be associated with guilt, and any indication of this should be mentioned to the physician. Bargaining can have a positive effect. It may give the client the hope and stamina to reach a desired goal. It is OK to mourn and cry. Allow for silences.

Depression

The dying client's body is deteriorating, sometimes rapidly; financial burdens are increasing; pain is unbearable; and relationships are severed. All can lead to depression. The dying are losing everything and everyone they love. Dying may be a time of tears, and crying may allow relief. Professionals who are happy, loud, and reassuring will not provide much help to depressed clients. Clients may need to express their sorrow to someone, or merely have someone close. They may have little need for words in this stage. Simple tasks may be impossible. Helplessness is real.

Acceptance

The final but perhaps not lasting stage is when clients are accepting of their fate. They usually are tired, weak, and able to sleep. They are not necessarily happy, but rather at peace. Professionals will be aware that clients may prefer to be left alone and not bothered with world events or family problems. Family members usually require more help, understanding, and support than clients in this stage. Touching and the use of silence may prove useful.

▚▚▚ HOSPICE

Dictionaries define the term *hospice* as "a lodging for travelers or young persons, especially when maintained by a religious order." The term later was used to describe lodging for dying clients. The first such hospice, Saint Christopher's, was formed by Cecily Saunders in London in 1965. Since then, the hospice concept has expanded throughout the United States.

Hospices provide care of the terminally ill at home, in a hospital, or in a special facility. The main objective of care is to make clients comfortable,

UNIFORM ANATOMICAL GIFT ACT

The legal definition of death is particularly important in the area of organ transplants. Under the old definitions, a surgeon removing a vital organ from a body still breathing and pulsating could technically be guilty of homicide. Many states, however, have adopted legislation making such actions possible. All 50 states have some form of the Uniform Anatomical Gift Act. Persons 18 years or older and of sound mind may make a gift of all or any part of their body to the following persons for the following purposes:

1. To any hospital, surgeon, or physician for medical or dental education, research, advancement of medical or dental science, therapy, or transplantation
2. To any accredited medical or dental school, college, or university for education, research, advancement of medical or dental science, or therapy
3. To any organ bank or storage facility, for medical or dental education, research, advancement of medical or dental science, therapy, or transplantation
4. To any specified individual for therapy or transplantation needed by him or her

The gift may be made by a provision in a will or by signing, in the presence of two witnesses, a card. The card is generally carried with the person at all times.[5] The latter method is the best because the living will may not be readily available until it is too late for donation of organs or tissues. Donated organs may include heart, lung, kidney, pancreas, liver, and intestine; tissue includes eyes, skin, bone, heart valves, veins, and tendons.

It is illegal to sell body parts in this country; however, the practice is common in developing countries. There is no cost to the family of the donor. Generally, there is no cost for later cremation or burial of the body parts.

Persons may place conditions on their organ donation. If a relative opposes the donation, most physicians and hospitals would not insist on the transplant. Donors are carefully screened before their body parts are used. The physician and hospital may be found negligent, so they must have strict standards for donor screening. Refer to Appendix II for a sample of the Uniform Donor Card.

Ethical issues include the following: What method is used to determine death in your state, and is it identified in the Uniform Anatomical Gift Act? The act is vague and does not specify the definition of death. Is dead really dead? Cultural differences exist, as well as religious differences in organ and tissue donation. For example, the Hmoges immigrant from Southeast Asia may believe that organ donation prevents the person from

"at home," and close to family. Treatments such as cardiopulmonary resuscitation, intravenous therapy, nasogastric tubes, and antibiotics are discouraged. Treatments are given in light of the client's personal and social circumstances.

The hospice staff attempts to create a positive atmosphere. Death is seen as "all right." A balance is kept between human needs and medical needs. Children are encouraged to be in the hospice as a reminder that life is an ongoing process. Clients might share a cup of tea with staff and each other rather than receiving an intravenous solution during their last hours.

An advantage the hospice offers is staff members who are experienced and want to care for the dying. Its services are provided only to the dying, and death is managed with dignity. The expense is generally less than acute care costs, and some insurance companies cover the costs. The dying client is not isolated behind curtains but rather is surrounded by others. An empty bed remains empty for at least 24 hours to allow adjustment by everyone. In addition, survivors are helped to deal with the death. If the hospice care is at home, clients are in familiar surroundings, have their favorite food, and are close to loved ones.

The hospice does have disadvantages. One problem is whether family members, with a hospice's help, can handle the care at home. It may be too much, physically and emotionally. Also, what about dying clients? Are they comfortable with the kind of care they receive in the hospice? Do they need or want more? Are they comfortable in dealing with death? We may be conditioned to expect dying clients to be in hospitals, not homes. One research study indicated that 80 percent of relatives preferred to have their terminally ill loved ones die in the hospital, whereas 80 percent of dying clients said they preferred to die at home.[2]

Vignette 13

When executing a living will of a 76-year-old man who has been advised to have kidney dialysis, whose authority is paramount when there is disagreement among the nephrologist, the primary care physician, the client, and the family?

Later the same client is on the dialysis machine, and wants to discontinue the machine against the advice of the nephrologist. Has the authority changed?

Would the authority change in either of the two preceding situations if dialysis is performed while the client is a hospital inpatient as opposed to a client in a dialysis center?

ASSISTED SUICIDE

Questions arise about whether physician-assisted suicide or euthanasia should be endorsed. Are the two similar, or are they different enough that the arguments for one do not apply to the other? It is physician-assisted suicide when the physician gives a client a lethal dose of medication so that the client can self-administer the medication; it is active euthanasia when a physician administers a lethal dose to the client. In either case of physician-assisted suicide or euthanasia, the physician is active and involved; however, in both cases the client decides whether to ask for the medication. The client makes the choices in dying. In physician-assisted suicide, the client acts last, whereas in active euthanasia, the physician acts last.[3]

Just as California and Washington were forerunners with their living wills and natural death laws, they were forerunners in seeking legislation that would give people the option to seek "aid in dying from physicians to end life in a dignified, painless and humane manner." Such proposed laws are much broader in their scope than any living will or physicians' directive. One example is Washington Initiative 119, which was defeated by the voters. This proposed law would in effect have legalized active euthanasia. The text of the initiative specifically stated that the legislation should not be "construed to condone, authorize, or approve mercy killing," and the proposed law did not obligate any physician or health care institution to comply with a client's request for aid in dying. The initiative did propose, however, that (1) physicians who provide aid in dying would be immune from prosecution for criminal or unprofessional conduct and (2) physicians or facilities that did not choose to comply with such a client request must make a "good faith effort" to transfer the client to a physician or to another facility that will carry out the "medical service."[4]

In 1994 Oregon became the third state, after Washington and California, to ask voters to pass an assisted-suicide measure. It passed, but was challenged by the courts. Then in 1997, the assisted suicide measure was reaffirmed by the Oregon voters. The measure is the nation's first to allow a physician to prescribe a lethal dose of medication when asked by a terminally ill client. The four safeguards for this measure are as follows: (1) The attending physician must truly convey informed consent, which must include all feasible opportunities such as pain management, hospice, and palliative care. (2) The attending physician diagnosis and prognosis must be confirmed by a consulting physician. The latter physician must verify that the client has made a voluntary and informed decision. (3) If either physician thinks the client might have depression that might impair judgment, a counseling session must be made. (4) The client making the request must do so both orally and in writing. The law details specific time lines and a waiting period for the client before receiving the lethal medication. The request must be witnessed by at least two people who can

verify the client's capacity to make a decision and that the decision is voluntary. Obviously, the measure poses valid concerns, but it is a testimony to the growing desire to have increased legal protection for options in dying.

CRITICAL THINKING EXERCISE

The U.S. Supreme Court recently ruled on Washington State's and New York State's assisted suicide laws. The nation's newspapers revealed that one justice's wife died of cancer, another justice is a cancer survivor, and a third justice's spouse works with cancer clients. They rejected the notion that assisted suicide is a fundamental liberty.

To ensure a person's ultimate choice, one physician has designed a procedure to help persons take their own lives. In June 1990 Dr. Jack Kevorkian allegedly used his "suicide machine" to assist in the death of 54-year-old Janet Adkins. Adkins was diagnosed as having Alzheimer's, a degenerative disease of the brain. She chose to end her life before she became incapacitated. Dr. Kevorkian was later arrested and charged with murder. The charge, however, was dismissed by the judge as insupportable. After allegedly assisting in the suicides of other people, however, Dr. Kevorkian has again been arrested and charged with murder. He has been ordered to stand trial again. At the date of publication, no guilty verdict is given.

On April 17, 1997, the U.S. Senate passed a bill barring the federal government from financing physician-assisted suicide. The vote was 99 to 0. The same measure previously cleared the House of Representatives by a vote of 398 to 16. Medicare and medicaid are prohibited from funding physician-assisted suicide. In June 1997, all nine Supreme Court justices refused to accept the fact that assisted suicide was a fundamental liberty for the terminally ill. Instead, they reinstated two state (Washington and New York) bans on the practice.

Legislation on physician-assisted suicide will be controversial, contradictory, confusing, and as emotional as legalization of abortion has been in the United States. Some questions to ponder on the subject include the following: What constitutes a lethal medication? How accurate can the prediction of death within 6 months be? Will a working definition of "terminal" be relaxed? Can physicians recognize depression or the inability of a client to make such a choice? What if the prescription fails to kill and the result debilitates the client? What happens to the client who asks for a lethal medication but is unable to administer it? Is that person's right less than the person who is able to administer the dose?

reincarnation and therefore also resists autopsy. Many Native Americans oppose organ donation because there is an enormous reverence for the body. It is both the residence and the manifestation of a person's essence. North American Quakers and Unitarians do not oppose organ donation or organ transplants. Autopsies are acceptable and may even be recommended. It is wise for health care professionals to know, understand, and appreciate cultural preferences.

AUTOPSY

An autopsy is an examination of a dead body to determine the cause of death. Statutes generally state who can authorize an autopsy. Coroners or medical examiners may give such authorization. Others include, in order of priority:

Authorization of Autopsy: Priority

1. The surviving spouse
2. Any child of the deceased who is 18 years of age or older
3. Any one of the parents of the deceased
4. Any adult sibling of the deceased

Autopsies may be complete or partial. In other words, a pathologist may perform an autopsy on the entire body and examine every part and organ or do an autopsy only of the thoracic cavity or the brain. The extremities rarely are involved unless indicated by trauma, prior surgical procedure, or vessel involvement. No parts of the body can be retained for any reason without consent from the family. If the autopsy is done properly and in a professional manner, the body can be viewed by survivors or at a funeral.

There are circumstances that require an autopsy. Autopsies offer valuable information for medical science and research. Survivors need to understand that knowledge gained from an autopsy may prevent another person from suffering similar circumstances.

THE ROLE OF THE PHYSICIAN AND AMBULATORY HEALTH CARE PROFESSIONALS

Clients with life-threatening illnesses have special needs. Their reactions in the dying process are expressed in their various stages or responses.

Regardless of how they present themselves, ambulatory health care employees need to assess where clients are and react openly to them.

One of the best ways to begin reacting to the dying client is to take a good, hard look at your own attitude toward pain, suffering, and dying. How can you be especially sensitive to these clients without being obvious? Will you be able to respond to the client's total needs rather than merely the client's medical needs? Can you be comfortable when clients cry, when clients laugh, when they joke about their condition?

Health care professionals need to be able to talk without fear or anxiety to provide information, and they must be able to listen to dying clients. For example, an ambulatory health care employee may be asked, "Will I get addicted to these narcotics?" If the employee's thoughts are, "The doctor never should have given you anything so powerful," this attitude will be sensed by the client.

Dying clients may exhibit negative or distasteful behaviors in the ambulatory health care setting. How will you handle it? Will you take it personally? Will you react negatively? Ignore it?

Clients may ask questions with hidden meaning or be truly blunt. Are you aware of nonverbal clues from clients? How will you react? What if you do not know any answers?

Dying clients may develop gross physical deformities or radically altered physical appearances. Will you be able to manage? If so, how?

Family and friends also will require your attention. What will you do when you reach the end of your rope and become too emotionally involved?

Client referrals may be made to counselors, pastors, attorneys, social workers, and hospice organizations. Do not fool yourself that you can be all things to all people. Health care professionals can feel free to refer.

After the client has died, physicians and employees will turn their focus to survivors. In telling survivors of the death, be honest and caring. It is a shocking and painful time for survivors, and they will need your utmost attention. Try to provide whatever support they need and remain with them until some family or close friends can come.

During the grieving process, survivors may call or come to your ambulatory health care setting for information or assistance. If you are unable to answer their questions or meet their needs, refer them to someone who can. Funeral directors and the clergy offer valuable help in planning the funeral, answering questions about the human remains, and helping survivors through the grieving process. Organizations such as Compassionate Friends (parents and family who have lost a child) and groups for widows or widowers can be recommended, if appropriate.

Children and death pose sensitive situations. The death of a child is a profound emotional experience for everyone, especially family. Explaining death to a child is also difficult. The age and maturity of children need to be taken into consideration. Children deserve the same honesty as an adult and need to be told that sorrow is acceptable and crying is okay. Reassure children that death is in no way their fault. Using a phrase such as "God took your daddy away" may cause the child to blame God. Follow the lead of children in their questions, and tell children you do not have all the answers. Memories should be cherished and encouraged. Children require the same ritual and sorrow that other family members go through.

Volumes have been written in the past decade on the subject of dying and death. The information in this chapter only highlights the areas that seem most appropriate for the ambulatory health care employee. See the Bibliography for further reference.

REFERENCES

1. Smith, JK: Free Fall. Judson, Valley Forge, Pa, 1975, p 7.
2. Barnard, C: Good Life. Good Death. Prentice-Hall, Englewood Cliffs, NJ, 1980, p 21.
3. Brock, DW: Voluntary active euthanasia. Hastings Cent Rep 22(2):10, 1992.
4. Campbell, CS: To die in Washington. Hastings Cent Rep 21(2):3, 1991.
5. Annas, GJ, Glantz, LH, and Katz, BF: The Rights of Doctors, Nurses and Allied Health Professionals. Avon Books, New York, 1981, p 228.

BIBLIOGRAPHY

Annas, GJ: Death by prescription: The Oregon initiative. N Engl J Med 331:1240, 1994.
Colen, BD: Organ concert. Time 148(14):70, 1996.
Furrow, BR, et al: Health Law. West, St Paul, Minn, 1995.
Gianelli, DM: Oregon voters face 'Rx-only' suicide initiative. American Medical News 12 Sept 1994.
Irish, DP, Lundquist, F, and Nelson, VJ: Ethnic Variations in Dying, Death, and Grief: Diversity in Universality. Taylor and Francis, Washington, DC, 1993.
Kubler-Ross, E: On Death and Dying. Macmillan, New York, 1972.
Senate votes to bar funds for suicides. Los Angeles Times April 17, 1997.

Discussion Questions

1. *Are there any generalizations on death that you might add to the authors'? Any you might delete? Which ones most likely would describe you?*

2. *Describe some problems faced by family members in a long-term illness.*

3. *Does the allocation of scarce medical resources influence the care given to someone who is dying?*

4. *List Kubler-Ross's five stages of dying and give an example of each.*

5. *A client leaves the ambulatory health care setting and says to the receptionist, "I know I am dying. You people are lying to me." What is your response?*

6. *Would you prefer to die in a hospice or a hospital? Justify your answer.*

7. *Enter into a discussion wherein you identify and discuss reasons why physician-assisted suicide meets with so much controversy. Do you agree or disagree?*

8. *Would you donate your organs or tissues? If so, which ones? If not, explain.*

9. *Under what circumstances might physicians decide not to tell clients they are dying?*

10. *What considerations are taken into account when telling a child about death?*

11. *Why might an autopsy be helpful? Why might one be refused?*

12. *What have you done to prepare for your own death? Do you have a will? Have you planned for your family? Have you made any decisions that should be shared with legal counsel or physicians?*

13. *Refer to Ted's case in Chapter 16. Could Ted's inability to respond to the nephrologist's question about dialysis imply that he had changed his mind regarding heroic measures? Who would be the best person to determine this?*

Have a Care!

LEARNING OBJECTIVES

Upon successful completion of this chapter, you will:

1. Cry.
2. Laugh.
3. Experience a client's dilemma in the ambulatory health care setting.
4. Become a little more human.

I am a patient with an appointment to see your physician at 10:30 AM today. It is early December.

I hurt. I can't function at home. I can't function at work. The pain in my back is so bad I can't lift my 5-month-old infant. It hurts to shower and turn the steering wheel of the car. I have to go to bed before my husband and then I can't move. The spasms are terrifying. They wake me.

I am so tired. I have no energy. I'm not really afraid. I trust the doctor. I know he'll find out what is wrong, fix it, and I'll be back to normal.

I'm taking time from work to be here. It is inconvenient, but I can do it. No one will do my job while I'm gone; it will wait for my return. It has to be done. I expect action today, though. I don't want sympathy.

I'm glad I don't have to wait long in your ambulatory health care setting. The pain is a little less; the psychologic release from knowing I'll soon be better is addicting. But I put up a front, too. I can't cry or tell the doctor how bad the pain really is. The office greeting is cheerful, but I could use some help with my clothes. I can hardly get them off. The bra is terrible, and the pantyhose are worse.

Your physician is quiet, professional, and concerned. I feel better just seeing him. His smile is warm. I can tell he cares. The examination is not too difficult. He finally says, "It looks serious. We have to run a lot of tests. It is going to take time to get to the bottom of this." Laboratory tests and x-rays are ordered. Any physical activity is allowed until it causes pain. I don't tell him how hard that will be. He tells me to bring my husband with me the next visit. I'm instructed to get dressed and go to the laboratory. The awful bra and pantyhose again, and it hurts to tie my shoes.

The atmosphere is sterile in the laboratory—cool and too professional. My mind is racing while I wait. I'm in torment. "What is it? What about my baby? Will I be able to take care of her? I've waited 36 years for her. Am I going to be a burden?"

The laboratory technician withdraws the blood, and I give the laboratory a urine specimen. The awful pantyhose again! "Collect a 24-hour urine." They hand me this weird antifreeze-like container with an opening like a vinegar bottle. It is white and has large black letters, "For 24-Hour Urine Only." I also am told to collect some feces. I'm handed three unfolded cardboard containers and some tiny spatulas. No instructions. I can leave with the antifreeze container and all!

As I leave, I wonder, how long do I wait? When will I know? I'm exhausted. I want to get home and see my husband. I need to talk to someone. Oh, the pain is bad. I hurt.

* * *

A telephone call a week later from your physician tells me the progress of the tests, but no indication of a diagnosis. He is very general in his conversation.

Christmas is a blur. There is no change in my condition. Questions from family and friends are no help. They don't understand. Neither do I. I hide my true feelings.

* * *

I'm back in your office a few weeks later with my husband. He had to take time from work. The receptionist seems surprised that my husband is with me. I wonder if she thinks I can't handle this. Well, I can't!

The consultation is hard. Your physician is open and honest. He tells us that a bone disease is rampant. It is a metabolic bone disorder. I hear him tell my husband that I can have no physical activity. I must take off work. I cannot drive. To fall would be disastrous. My bones are like a loaf of bread. "You know what a loaf of bread is like when it is smashed." I cannot lift anything, even my baby. I'm not supposed to bend over. My husband asks, "Should we have outside help come into the home?" The doctor says, "Yes." I immediately think about the cost. The doctor tells me what kind of medications I'll be taking. But the final blow is his words that something else is wrong. He hopes more tests will reveal what.

* * *

A month passes. I'm having such a hard time having someone do my work. I find a replacement at my job. I don't ask for help easily. It is so hard to be inactive. I can't get my own groceries. I'm terrified of falling. I can't vacuum my floors. I can't lift my baby to change her. If she cries, I can't pick her up. Having someone else do those things I'm supposed to do is terrible. And when no one is looking, I do lift her. I do carry her. And I do damage my body. This creates conflict with my husband. Life is not good.

During this time, there are more tests and more referrals. More doctors. I feel like a "nothing." I feel inhuman. The worst tests are the intestinal or small bowel biopsies. Your physician tells me that they put a tube in my mouth and pass it through to the small intestine. It is painless and won't take very long.

My husband takes me to the test and is told I'll be finished in about $1\frac{1}{2}$ hours. They will call him. In the examination room, I'm partially disrobed and I put on a $\frac{3}{4}$-length gown that opens down the back. I can keep my slacks and shoes on. The gastroenterologist passed the tube through my mouth into my stomach. There is no pain, but it is awful. I gag over and over again. I must try not to. I tell myself to breathe slowly; concentrate on not vomiting. When the gastroenterologist finishes, the LPN says, "Let's go to x-ray."

To my horror, she hands me a box of tissues and an emesis basin, drapes my coat over my shoulders, takes my elbow, and says, "Be careful not to fall." I bite on the tube in my mouth and try to stabilize it with my free hand as we walk through a large, crowded reception area, out the front door, and across two office parking lots covered with early morning frost. While I am still in disbelief, we walk into the lowest floor of a multiple-office building where the x-ray receptionist tells us the radiologist is still at the hospital making rounds. I snarl through my teeth, "Get that doctor here now."

In the x-ray waiting area, I sit for 30 minutes, still trying not to gag. The tears come, first haltingly, then freely. The saliva flows from my mouth and nose. I'm finally able to get a hold of myself. I stop crying. I don't want to ruin the test. Finally the doctor appears. He looks at me. In my revulsion at the situation and him, I whisper, "You son of a—!" His response is, "What's wrong with you?" How can I tell him? I still have the tube in my mouth. He checks the placement of the tube in the small intestine several different times. When he verifies that it is in place, he calls another LPN to take me back. Over the same route. I pray to God no one recognizes me. I am in a state of shock about my circumstances.

Upon returning, the biopsy is taken. The doctor pulls the tube; I sigh with relief. In a few minutes, he turns to me and says, "We didn't get it." The instrument to snatch a piece of the intestinal wall didn't grab properly. The same procedure must be done again. The tube goes back in, across the parking lots, check the tube, back across the parking lots. This time, the biopsy is successful!

My husband is trying to call the office and wondering what has happened. They tell him only that there is a problem. He's not allowed to speak to anyone else. Four and one-half hours later, they call to tell him I'm finished.

* * *

Ten years have passed. I'm now living with the metabolic bone disorder, which is somewhat improved. I have an intestinal malabsorption problem that is totally controlled by diet. My activities are somewhat limited. I cannot lift anything heavy or participate in any sport other than swimming, but I no longer need help at home. I must take much medication, some of it experimental, and I'm 4 inches shorter.

I have a hearing loss that requires the use of hearing aids. Speech sounds are distorted. Pain is always with me. I am afraid I will someday be confined to a wheelchair and fear that I might have to quit work. I wonder why my body has to be so "unusual."

On good days, I remind myself that I must live in the here and now. I continue my teaching with urgency. I am glad that I can handle pain. I thank God daily for my coauthor, who brings out the best in me. (Someday I will be as short as she.) I practice a healthful lifestyle and willingly share my sense of humor. I enjoy life to the very fullest. My family and friends give me strength. I've loved being an author of this book.

* * *

Now it's almost 20 years since the first edition of this book.

Life changes in many ways. My dearest daughter and only born goes to college, leaving an emptiness filled with getting to reknow why my husband and I married in the first place! How things change. . . . Even though the nest is empty and I experience all the emotions that go along with that, I am eternally grateful that I have met and passed a milestone in my daughter's life that I once thought I might never see.

My health is not as good as it used to be—that's what aging does and what happens when you are chronically ill. My ribs sit within my pelvis and sometimes when the bones rub, it hurts beyond belief. Yes, the rehab physician fits me with a brace but it doesn't work because my height changes drastically as the day progresses—no brace can adjust to those changes! Even today my dear friend and I measured ourselves against the wall! She used to joke that one day we'll both shop in petites and as I'm measuring 5'5" instead of 5'10", we're also laughing that she's just 5'instead of 5'2"!

Pain is ever present. On a scale of 1 to 10 most days it ranges between a 3 and an 8; some days it's a 20, but I refuse to suffer. I choose to live life to its fullest. I choose not to complain or let any person dare even guess what's going on in my life. Rapture is my family, my writing with my coauthor and best-est friend, and adding balance to my life. The albatross around my neck is when I work too hard, when I ignore the increasing pain, when I won't ask for the bellman to take my bags out of the trunk of my car, and when I walk across campus with too many books.

My deafness increases, but dear friends and family make sure I don't miss anything important. I continue to seek treatment from specialists. They care and provide excellent management. I easily discriminate between those who care and those who don't. It's easy to feel and see the difference. It's those that provide me the compassion and the professional care that count. The "please," the "thank you," the "good job, Marti!"

My hope had been that with increased awareness of client needs in health care, the importance of therapeutic communication with the client, and the high demands for prevention, the health care professionals would never be as bad as the ones I first experienced, but occasionally they are still there.

Recently, when I chose to have a totally independent second opinion, the physician ordered a back x-ray. I entered the x-ray room and positioned myself as instructed. The technician said in a demeaning tone, "You're not standing up straight." I replied, "I am!" She said, "Nobody's that crooked," and she attempted to straighten my body. It didn't work. She was angry. "If we don't get it right this time, we'll have to do it over." I was shocked. I felt rage, anger, embarrassment, shame, and disgust. I wanted to do what I was told.

My sense of humor sees me through. Recalling situations such as the back x-ray, I contemplate how I could "get even" or "get ahead!" My family and friends are my strength. They know who I am. They accept me as I am. I can be me. It's OK to be the Velveteen Rabbit. My dearest friend is always there, anticipating, understanding, and so very caring. She teaches me about life by her mentoring. She's learned to carry two purses, two bags, and she eats my rice crackers. Life is good!

I'll work a few more years, then hopefully do what comes naturally. . . .

We share this with you because we care. We hope by sharing, by being transparent, that we give you permission and enable you to be transparent. Share your compassion. Model how health care professionals should act. Let us remind you again, please remember to be loving, to be gracious, to be human, and to be able to put yourself in the place of your clients. Try to remember that the client is more than a person with an illness. Clients are persons with responsibilities, with families, and with personal and emotional needs. Professionals care for the whole person. Have a care!

Discussion Questions

1. *Was any health professional a "listener" for this person?*
2. *What kind of nonverbal messages did the client send?*
3. *What positive forms of conduct and courtesy were shown to the client?*

4. *What negative forms of conduct and courtesy were shown to the client?*

5. *What could you have done as a receptionist, as a nurse, as a laboratory or x-ray technician, as a medical assistant, and as a physician?*

6. *Examine the value of truly revealing yourself to another.*

Epilogue

This book has been written for you: you who are employed in ambulatory health care; you who are students in medical assisting or other health care programs in schools, colleges, and universities; you who are physicians spending the major portion of your working day in your ambulatory health care setting treating clients.

We have cared for your clients at home; we have worked in your ambulatory health care settings and hospitals; we have taught in your classes; we have been your clients. We know the great responsibility you carry as employees; we delight in your excitement about preparing yourself to work for physicians; we appreciate your role as physicians and business managers in the ambulatory health care setting.

We have not tried to be your legal counsel; we have not attempted to know all of your state's statutes; we have not wanted to be your conscience in the complex world of bioethics.

We hope we have been your guide; we hope we have stimulated your interest in the law; we hope we have aroused your compassion and empathy for any person struggling for answers in any of the issues in bioethics; we hope you have a helpful reference for ambulatory health care; please buy another 100,000 copies!

We have laughed; we have cried; our demanding work schedules require that we retreat to comfortable surroundings away from home to write, rewrite, research, and cogitate. We have deepened our knowledge base; our compassionate tendency has broadened in scope; neither of us tolerates less than caring, professional treatment by any health care professional. We demand the same from our students.

The first edition in its infancy created a fine friendship. The maturity reflected in this fourth edition is seen also in the breadth and depth of our continuing friendship. Even in our differences and disagreements, the final product is whole because we complete each other. May you never dim your light to the mediocrity of health care. And may you, too, find such a friend to heal yourself.

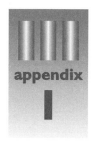

Codes of Ethics

▰▰▰ THE HIPPOCRATIC OATH*

I swear by Apollo Physician and Aslepius and Hygieia and Panaceia and all the gods and goddesses, making them my witnesses, that I will fulfil according to my ability and judgment this oath and this covenant:

To hold him who has taught me this art as equal to my parents and to live my life in partnership with him, and if he is in need of money to give him a share of mine, and to regard his offspring as equal to my brothers in male lineage and to teach them this art if they desire to learn it without fee and covenant; to give a share of precepts and oral instruction and all the other learning to my sons and to the sons of him who has instructed me and to pupils who have signed the covenant and have taken an oath according to the medical law, but to no one else.

I will apply dietetic measures for the benefit of the sick according to my ability and judgment; I will keep them from harm and injustice.

I will neither give a deadly drug to anybody if asked for it, nor will I make a suggestion to this effect. Similarly I will not give to a woman an abortive remedy. In purity and holiness I will guard my life and my art.

I will not use the knife, not even on sufferers from stone, but will withdraw in favor of such men as are engaged in this work.

Whatever houses I may visit, I will come for the benefit of the sick, remaining free of all intentional injustice, of all mischief and in particular of sexual relations with both female and male persons, be they free or slaves.

What I may see or hear in the course of the treatment or even outside of the treatment in regard to the life of men, which on no account one must spread abroad, I will keep to myself holding such things shameful to be spoken about.

---

*From Ludwig, E: The Hippocratic oath. In Oswei, T, and Temkin, CL (eds): Ancient Medicine. Johns Hopkins University Press, Baltimore, 1967, with permission.

If I fulfil this oath and do not violate it, may it be granted to me to enjoy life and art, being honored with fame among all men for all time to come; if I transgress it and swear falsely, may the opposite of all this be my lot.

THE GENEVA CONVENTION CODE OF MEDICAL ETHICS*

I solemnly pledge myself to consecrate my life to the service of humanity;

I will give to my teachers the respect and gratitude which is their due;

I will practice my profession with conscience and dignity;

The health of my patient will be my first consideration;

I will respect the secrets which are confided in me;

I will maintain by all means in my power, the honour, and the noble traditions of the medical profession;

My colleagues will be my brothers;

I will not permit considerations of religion, nationality, race, party politics, or social standing to intervene between my duty and my patient.

I will maintain the utmost respect for human life from the time of conception; even under threat, I will not use my medical knowledge contrary to the laws of humanity.

I make these promises solemnly, freely, and upon my honour.

---

*From the World Medical Association, Adopted by the World Medical Association in 1949, with permission.

■ THE NUREMBERG CODE*

The great weight of the evidence before us is to the effect that certain types of medical experiments on human beings, when kept within reasonably well-defined bounds, conform to the ethics of the medical profession generally. The protagonists of the practice of human experimentation justify their views on the basis that such experiments yield results for the good of society that are unprocurable by other methods or means of study. All agree, however, that certain basic principles must be observed in order to satisfy moral, ethical, and legal concepts.

1. The voluntary consent of the human subject is absolutely essential.

This means that the person involved should have legal capacity to give consent; should be so situated as to be able to exercise free power of choice, without the intervention of any element of force, fraud, deceit, duress, overreaching, or other ulterior form of constraint or coercion; and should have sufficient knowledge and comprehension of the elements of the subject matter involved as to enable him to make an understanding and enlightened decision. This latter element requires that before the acceptance of an affirmative decision by the experimental subject there should be made known to him the nature, duration, and purpose of the experiment; the method and means by which it is to be conducted; all inconveniences and hazards reasonably to be expected; and the effects upon his health or person which may possibly come from his participation in the experiment.

The duty and responsibility for ascertaining the quality of the consent rests upon each individual who initiates, directs, or engages in the experiment. It is a personal duty and responsibility which may not be delegated to another with impunity.

2. The experiment should be such as to yield fruitful results for the good of society, unprocurable by other methods or means of study, and not random and unnecessary in nature.
3. The experiment should be so designed and based on the results of animal experimentation and a knowledge of the natural history of the disease or other problem under study that the anticipated results will justify the performance of the experiment.
4. The experiment should be so conducted as to avoid all unnecessary physical and mental suffering and injury.
5. No experiment should be conducted where there is an a priori reason to believe that death or disabling injury will occur; except where the experimental physicians also serve as subjects.

---

*From Trials of War Criminals before the Nuremberg Military Tribunals under Control Council Law No. 10, Vol. II, Nuremberg, October 1946 to April 1949.

6. The degree of risk to be taken should never exceed that determined by the humanitarian importance of the problem to be solved by the experiment.
7. Proper preparations should be made and adequate facilities provided to protect the experimental subject against even remote possibilities of injury, disability, or death.
8. The experiment should be conducted only by scientifically qualified persons. The highest degree of skill and care should be required through all stages of the experiment of those who conduct or engage in the experiment.
9. During the course of the experiment, the human subject should be at liberty to bring the experiment to an end if he has reached the physical or mental state where continuation of the experiment seems to him to be impossible.
10. During the course of the experiment, the scientist in charge must be prepared to terminate the experiment at any stage, if he has probable cause to believe, in the exercise of the good faith, superior skill and careful judgment required of him that a continuation of the experiment is likely to result in injury, disability, or death to the experimental subject.

▇ DECLARATION OF HELSINKI*— RECOMMENDATIONS GUIDING MEDICAL DOCTORS IN BIOMEDICAL RESEARCH INVOLVING HUMAN SERVICES, WORLD MEDICAL ASSOCIATION

Introduction

It is the mission of the medical doctor to safeguard the health of the people. His or her knowledge and conscience are dedicated to the fulfillment of this mission.

The Declaration of Geneva of the World Medical Association binds the doctor with the words. "The health of my patient will be my first consideration"; the International Code of Medical Ethics declares that, "Any act or advice which could weaken physical or mental resistance of a human being may be used only in his interest."

The purpose of biomedical research involving human subjects must be to improve diagnostic, therapeutic, and prophylactic procedures and the understanding of the etiology and pathogenesis of disease.

In current medical practice, most diagnostic, therapeutic, or prophylactic procedures involve hazards. This applies a fortiori to biomedical research.

Medical progress is based on research which ultimately must rest in part on experimentation involving human subjects.

In the field of biomedical research, a fundamental distinction must be recognized between medical research in which the aim is essentially diagnostic or therapeutic for a patient, and medical research, the essential object of which is purely scientific and without direct diagnostic or therapeutic value to the person subjected to the research.

Special caution must be exercised in the conduct of research which may affect the environment, and the welfare of animals used for research must be respected.

Because it is essential that the results of laboratory experiments be applied to human beings to further scientific knowledge and to help suffering humanity, the World Medical Association has prepared the following recommendations as a guide to every doctor in biomedical research involving human subjects. They should be kept under review in the future. It must be stressed that the standards as drafted are only a guide to physicians all over the world. Doctors are not relieved from criminal, civil, and ethical responsibilities under the laws of their own countries.

---

*From the World Medical Association, Inc.: Declaration of Helsinki, revised edition, with permission. Adopted by the 18th World Medical Assembly, Helsinki, Finland, 1964, and revised by the 29th World Medical Assembly, Tokyo, Japan, October 1975.

I. Basic Principles

1. Biomedical research involving human subjects must conform to generally accepted scientific principles and should be based on adequately performed laboratory and animal experimentation and on a thorough knowledge of the scientific literature.

2. The design and performance of each experimental procedure involving human subjects should be clearly formulated in an experimental protocol which should be transmitted to a specially appointed independent committee for consideration, comment, and guidance.

3. Biomedical research involving human subjects should be conducted only by scientifically qualified persons and under the supervision of a clinically competent medical person. The responsibility for the human subject must always rest with a medically qualified person and never rest on the subject of research, even though the subject has given his or her consent.

4. Biomedical research involving human subjects cannot legitimately be carried out unless the importance of the objective is in proportion to the inherent risk to the subject.

5. Every biomedical research project involving human subjects should be preceded by careful assessment of predictable risks in comparison with foreseeable benefits to the subjects or to others. Concern for the interests of the subject must always prevail over the interests of science and society.

6. The right of the research subject to safeguard his or her integrity must always be respected. Every precaution should be taken to respect the privacy of the subject and to minimize the impact of the study on the subject's physical and mental integrity and on the personality of the subject.

7. Doctors should abstain from engaging in research projects involving human subjects unless they are satisfied that the hazards involved are believed to be predictable. Doctors should cease any investigation if the hazards are found to outweigh the potential benefits.

8. In publication of the results of his or her research, the doctor is obliged to preserve the accuracy of the results. Reports of experimentation not in accordance with the principles laid down in this Declaration should not be accepted for publication.

9. In any research on human beings, each potential subject must be adequately informed of the aims, methods, anticipated benefits and potential hazards of the study, and the discomfort it may entail. He or she should be informed that he or she is at liberty to abstain from participation in the study and that he or she is free to withdraw his or her consent to participation at any time. The doctor should then obtain the subject's freely given informed consent, preferably in writing.

10. When obtaining informed consent for the research project, the doctor should be particularly cautious if the subject is in a dependent relationship to him or her or may consent under duress. In that case the informed consent should be obtained by a doctor who is not engaged in the investigation and who is completely independent of this official relationship.

11. In case of legal incompetence, informed consent should be obtained from the legal guardian in accordance with national legislation. Where physical or mental incapacity makes it impossible to obtain informed consent, or when the subject is a minor, permission from the responsible relative replaces that of the subject in accordance with national legislation.

12. The research protocol should always contain a statement of the ethical considerations involved and should indicate that the principles enunciated in the present Declaration are complied with.

II. Medical Research Combined with Professional Care (Clinical Research)

1. In the treatment of the sick person, the doctor must be free to use a new diagnostic and therapeutic measure, if in his or her judgment it offers hope of saving life, reestablishing health, or alleviating suffering.

2. The potential benefits, hazards, and discomfort of a new method should be weighed against the advantages of the best current diagnostic and therapeutic methods.

3. In any medical study, every patient including those of a control group, if any should be assured of the best proven diagnostic and therapeutic method.

4. The refusal of the patient to participate in a study must never interfere with the doctor/patient relationship.

5. If the doctor considers it essential not to obtain informed consent, the specific reasons for this proposal should be stated in the experimental protocol for transmission to the independent committee. (I, 2)

6. The doctor can combine medical research with professional care, the objective being the acquisition of new medical knowledge, only to the extent that medical research is justified by its potential diagnostic or therapeutic value for the patient.

III. Nontherapeutic Biomedical Research Involving Human Subjects (Nonclinical Biomedical Research)

1. In the purely scientific application of medical research carried out on a human being, it is the duty of the doctor to remain the protec-

tor of life and health of that person on whom biomedical research is being carried out.

2. The subjects should be volunteers either healthy persons or patients for whom the experimental design is not related to the patient's illness.

3. The investigator or the investigating team should discontinue the research if in his/her or their judgment it may, if continued, be harmful to the individual.

4. In research on man, the interest of science and society should never take precedence over considerations related to the well-being of the subject.

CODES FOR NURSES*

Ethical Concepts Applied to Nursing

The fundamental responsibility of the nurse is fourfold: to promote health, to prevent illness, to restore health, and to alleviate suffering.

The need for nursing is universal. Inherent in nursing is respect for life, dignity, and rights of man. It is unrestricted by considerations of nationality, race, creed, color, age, sex, politics, or social status. Nurses render health services to the individual, the family, and the community and coordinate their services with those of related groups.

Nurses and People

The nurse's primary responsibility is to those people who require nursing care.

The nurse, in providing care, promotes an environment in which the values, customs, and spiritual beliefs of the individual are respected.

The nurse holds in confidence personal information and uses judgment in sharing this information.

Nurses and Practice

The nurse carries personal responsibility for nursing practice and for maintaining competence by continual learning.

The nurse maintains the highest standards of nursing care possible within the reality of a specific situation.

The nurse uses judgment in relation to individual competence when accepting the delegating responsibilities.

The nurse when acting in a professional capacity should at all times maintain standards of personal conduct which reflect credit upon the profession.

Nurses and Society

The nurse shares with other citizens the responsibility for initiating and supporting action to meet the health and social needs of the public.

Nurses and Co-Workers

The nurse sustains a cooperative relationship with co-workers in nursing and other fields.

The nurse takes appropriate action to safeguard the individual when his care is endangered by a co-worker or any other person.

---

*From the International Council of Nurses, Geneva, Switzerland, with permission. The Code for Nurses, as printed here, was produced by the Professional Services Committee and adopted by the ICN Council of National Representatives in Mexico City in May 1973.

Nurses and the Profession

The nurse plays the major role in determining and implementing desirable standards of nursing practice and nursing education.

The nurse is active in developing a core of professional knowledge.

The nurse, acting through the professional organization, participates in establishing and maintaining equitable social and economic working conditions in nursing.

▬ AMERICAN ASSOCIATION OF MEDICAL ASSISTANTS

The Code of Ethics of AAMA shall set forth principles of ethical and moral conduct as they relate to the medical profession and the particular practice of medical assisting.

Members of AAMA dedicated to the conscientious pursuit of their profession, and thus desiring to merit the high regard of the entire medical profession and the respect of the general public which they serve, do pledge themselves to strive always to:

A. Render service with full respect for the dignity of humanity;
B. Respect confidential information obtained through employment unless legally authorized or required by responsible performance of duty to divulge such information;
C. Uphold the honor and high principles of the profession and accept its disciplines;
D. Seek to continually improve the knowledge and skills of medical assistants for the benefit of patients and professional colleagues;
E. Participate in additional service activities aimed toward improving the health and well-being of the community.

Creed

I believe in the principles and purposes of the profession of medical assisting.

I endeavor to be more effective.
I aspire to render greater service.
I protect the confidence entrusted to me.
I am dedicated to the care and well-being of all people.
I am loyal to my employer.
I am true to the ethics of my profession.
I am strengthened by compassion, courage, and faith.

■ PRINCIPLES OF MEDICAL ETHICS: AMERICAN MEDICAL ASSOCIATION*

Preamble

The medical profession has long subscribed to a body of ethical statements developed primarily for the benefit of the patient. As a member of this profession, a physician must recognize responsibility not only to patients, but also to society, to other health professionals, and to self. The following Principles adopted by the American Medical Association are not laws, but standards of conduct which define the essentials of honorable behavior for the physician.

  I. A physician shall be dedicated to providing competent medical service with compassion and respect for human dignity.
 II. A physician shall deal honestly with patients and colleagues, and strive to expose those physicians deficient in character or competence, or who engage in fraud or deception.
III. A physician shall respect the law and also recognize a responsibility to seek changes in those requirements which are contrary to the best interests of the patient.
 IV. A physician shall respect the rights of patients, of colleagues, and of other health professionals, and shall safeguard patient confidences within the constraints of the law.
  V. A physician shall continue to study, apply, and advance scientific knowledge; make relevant information available to patients, colleagues, and the public; obtain consultation; and use the talents of other health professionals when indicated.
 VI. A physician shall, in the provision of appropriate patient care, except in emergencies, be free to choose whom to serve, with whom to associate, and the environment in which to provide medical services.
VII. A physician shall recognize a responsibility to participate in activities contributing to an improved community.

▆▆▆ A PATIENT'S BILL OF RIGHTS: AMERICAN HOSPITAL ASSOCIATION*

The American Hospital Association (AHA) Board of Trustees' Committee on Health Care for the Disadvantaged, which has been a consistent advocate on behalf of consumers of health care services, developed the Statement on a Patient's Bill of Rights, which was approved by the AHA House of Delegates February 6, 1973. The statement was published in several forms, one of which was the S74 leaflet in the Association's S series. The S74 leaflet is now superseded by this reprinting of the statement.

The American Hospital Association presents a Patient's Bill of Rights with the expectation that observance of these rights will contribute to more effective patient care and greater satisfaction for the patient, his physician, and the hospital organization. Further, the Association presents these rights in the expectation that they will be supported by the hospital on behalf of its patients, as an integral part of the healing process. It is recognized that a personal relationship between the physician and the patient is essential for the provision of proper medical care. The traditional physician/patient relationship takes on a new dimension when care is rendered within an organizational structure. Legal precedent has established that the institution itself also has a responsibility to the patient. It is in recognition of these factors that these rights are affirmed.

1. The patient has the right to considerate and respectful care.
2. The patient has the right to obtain from his physician complete current information concerning his diagnosis, treatment, and prognosis in terms the patient can be reasonably expected to understand. When it is not medically advisable to give such information to the patient, the information should be made available to an appropriate person in his behalf. He has the right to know, by name, the physician responsible for coordinating his care.
3. The patient has the right to receive from his physician information necessary to give informed consent prior to the start of any procedure and/or treatment. Except in emergencies, such information for informed consent should include but not necessarily be limited to the specific procedure and/or treatment, the medically significant risks involved, and the probable duration of incapacitation. Where medically significant alternatives for care or treatment exist, or when the patient requests information concerning medical alternatives, the patient has the right to such information. The patient also has the right to know the name of the person responsible for the procedures and/or treatment.

---

*From the American Hospital Association, copyright 1975, with permission.

4. The patient has the right to refuse treatment to the extent permitted by law and to be informed of the medical consequences of his action.

5. The patient has the right to every consideration of his privacy concerning his own medical care program. Case discussion, consultation, examination, and treatment are confidential and should be conducted discreetly. Those not directly involved in his care must have the permission of the patient to be present.

6. The patient has the right to expect that all communications and records pertaining to his care should be treated as confidential.

7. The patient has the right to expect that within its capacity a hospital must make reasonable response to the request of a patient for services. The hospital must provide evaluation, service, and/or referral as indicated by the urgency of the case. When medically permissible, a patient may be transferred to another facility only after he has received complete information and explanation concerning the needs for and alternatives to such a transfer. The institution to which the patient is to be transferred must first have accepted the patient for transfer.

8. The patient has the right to obtain information as to any relationship of his hospital to other health care and educational institutions insofar as his care is concerned. The patient has the right to obtain information as to the existence of any professional relationships among individuals, by name, who are treating him.

9. The patient has the right to be advised if the hospital proposes to engage in or perform human experimentation affecting his care or treatment. The patient has the right to refuse to participate in such research projects.

10. The patient has the right to expect reasonable continuity of care. He has the right to know in advance what appointment times and physicians are available and where. The patient has the right to expect that the hospital will provide a mechanism whereby he is informed by his physician or a delegate of the physician of the patient's continuing health care requirement following discharge.

11. The patient has the right to examine and receive an explanation of his bill regardless of source of payment.

12. The patient has the right to know what hospital rules and regulations apply to his conduct as a patient. No catalog of rights can guarantee for the patient the kind of treatment he has a right to expect. A hospital has many functions to perform, including the prevention and treatment of disease, the education of both health professionals and patients, and the conduct of clinical research. All these activities must be conducted with an overriding concern for the patient, and, above all, the recognition of his dignity as a human being. Success in achieving this recognition assures success in the defense of the right of the patient.

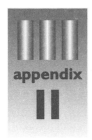

Sample Documents for Choices about Health Care, Life, and Death

▰▰▰ WASHINGTON STATE HEALTH CARE DIRECTIVE*

Directive made this _____ day of _____ (month, year).

I _____ , having the capacity to make health care decisions, willfully, and voluntarily make known my desire that my dying shall not be artificially prolonged under the circumstance set forth below, and do hereby declare that:

(a) If at any time I should be diagnosed in writing to be in a terminal condition by the attending physician or in a permanent unconscious condition by two physicians, and where the application of life-sustaining treatment would serve to artificially prolong the process of dying, I direct that such treatment be withheld or withdrawn and that I be permitted to die naturally. I understand by using this form that a terminal condition means an incurable and irreversible condition caused by injury, disease, or illness, that would within reasonable medical judgment cause death within a reasonable period of time in accordance with accepted medical standards, and where the application of life-sustaining treatment would serve only to prolong the process of dying. I further understand in using this form that a permanent unconscious condition means an incurable and irreversible condition in which I am medically assessed within reasonable medical judgment as having no reasonable probability of recovery from an irreversible coma or a persistent vegetative state.

(b) In such absence of my ability to give directions regarding the use of such life-sustaining treatment, it is my intention that this directive shall be honored by my family and physician(s) as the final expression of my legal

---

*From Chapter 98, Laws of 1992, Natural Death Act Revisions, Sec. 3. RCW 70.122.030. Effective date: 6/11/92.

right to refuse medical or surgical treatment, and I accept the consequences of such refusal. If another person is appointed to make these decisions for me, whether through a durable power of attorney or otherwise, I request that the person be guided by this directive and any other clear expression of my desires.

(c) If I am diagnosed to be in a terminal condition or in a permanent unconscious condition (check one):

I DO want to have artificially provided nutrition and hydration.

I DO NOT want to have artificially provided nutrition and hydration.

(d) If I have been diagnosed as pregnant and that diagnosis is known to my physician, this directive shall have no force or effect during the course of pregnancy.

(e) I understand the full import of this directive and I am emotionally and mentally capable to make the health care decisions contained in this directive.

(f) I understand that before I sign this directive, I can add to or delete from or otherwise change the wording of this directive and that I may add or delete from this directive at any time and that any changes shall be consistent with Washington state law or federal constitutional law to be legally valid.

(g) It is my wish that every part of this directive be fully implemented. If for any reason any part is held invalid, it is my wish that the remainder of my directive be implemented.

Signed _____
City, County, and State of Residence

The declarer has been personally known to me, and I believe him or her to be capable of making health care decisions.

Witness _____
Witness _____

WASHINGTON STATE DURABLE POWER OF ATTORNEY FOR HEALTH CARE*

I, _____, domiciled in the State of Washington, designate _____ as my attorney in fact, to act for me if I become incapacitated. I hereby revoke all health care powers of attorney previously granted by me.

1. Alternate Attorney in Fact. If for any reason _____ fails or ceases to act, I designate _____, then _____ as alternate attorneys in fact, to serve in the order named. An attorney in fact may resign by delivering written notice to that effect in recordable form, to an alternate, successor, or co-attorney in fact. In this Power of Attorney, the "attorney in fact" means the then-acting attorney in fact.

2. Power to Make Health Care Decisions. My attorney in fact shall have the right to make decisions and to give informed consent on my behalf as to my health care. To the extent permitted by law, this shall include but not be limited to, the right to consent to the withholding or withdrawal of life-sustaining procedures which would only prolong artificially the moment of my death and prevent me from dying naturally, in those circumstances where my physicians have determined (a) that I am in a comatose or persistent vegetative state from which there is no reasonable probability of my recovery or (b) that I have a terminal condition and my death is imminent unless, or even if, such life-sustaining procedures are utilized. I include in these life-sustaining procedures the artificial administration of food and fluids.

3. Effectiveness. This Power of Attorney shall become effective upon my incapacity. Incapacity shall include the inability to make health care decisions effectively for reasons such as mental illness, mental deficiency, incompetency, physical illness or disability, advanced age, chronic use of drugs or chronic intoxication. Incapacity may be determined (i) by court order or (ii) by a qualified regularly attending physician, whose affidavit in recordable form to that effect shall be conclusive of incapacity. An affidavit executed as described herein may be relied upon without inquiry by any person dealing with the attorney in fact.

4. Duration. This Power of Attorney becomes effective as provided in Section 3 and shall remain in effect to the fullest extent permitted by Chapter 11.94 of the Revised Code of Washington, or until revoked or terminated as provided in Section 5 or 6.

*From the Washington State Hospital Association, with permission.

5. Revocation. This Power of Attorney may be revoked, suspended, or terminated by written notice from me to the designated attorney in fact, and, if this power has been recorded, by recording the notice in the office where deeds are recorded for real estate located in _____ County, Washington.

6. Termination. If appointed, a guardian of my person may, with court approval, revoke, suspend, or terminate this Power of Attorney.

7. Reliance. Any person dealing with the attorney in fact shall be entitled to rely upon this Power of Attorney so long as the person with whom the attorney in fact was dealing, at the time of any act taken pursuant to this Power of Attorney, had neither actual knowledge nor written notice of any revocation, suspension, or termination of the Power of Attorney. Any action so taken, unless otherwise invalid or unenforceable, shall be binding on my heirs, devisees, legatees, or personal representatives.

8. Indemnity. My estate shall hold harmless and indemnify the attorney in fact from all liability for acts or omissions done in good faith.

9. Applicable Law. The internal law of the State of Washington shall govern this Power of Attorney.

10. Execution. This Power of Attorney is signed in duplicate on the _____ day of _____, to be effective as provided in Section 3.

Signed _____

Witness _____
Witness _____

I certify that I know or have satisfactory evidence that _____
_____ signed this instrument and acknowledged it to be a free and voluntary act for the uses and purposes mentioned in the instrument.

Date: _____   _____

■■■ UNIFORM DONOR CARD

In the hope that I may help others, I hereby make this anatomical gift, if medically acceptable, to take effect upon my death. The words and marks below indicate my desire to give: (please check one box only)

(a) _____ any needed organs or parts

(b) _____ only the following organs or parts (please specify)

_____

(c) _____ my whole body for anatomical study if needed

Limitations or special wishes if any:

_____

Signed by the donor and the following two witnesses in the presence of each other

Donor signature _____

Date of birth _____ Date signed _____

Witness _____
Witness _____

This is a legal document under the Uniform Anatomical Gift Act and should be carried on your person at all times.

Index

Note: Page numbers followed by "f" indicate illustrations; those followed by "t" indicate tables.

"at home," and close to family. Treatments such as cardiopulmonary resuscitation, intravenous therapy, nasogastric tubes, and antibiotics are discouraged. Treatments are given in light of the client's personal and social circumstances.

The hospice staff attempts to create a positive atmosphere. Death is seen as "all right." A balance is kept between human needs and medical needs. Children are encouraged to be in the hospice as a reminder that life is an ongoing process. Clients might share a cup of tea with staff and each other rather than receiving an intravenous solution during their last hours.

An advantage the hospice offers is staff members who are experienced and want to care for the dying. Its services are provided only to the dying, and death is managed with dignity. The expense is generally less than acute care costs, and some insurance companies cover the costs. The dying client is not isolated behind curtains but rather is surrounded by others. An empty bed remains empty for at least 24 hours to allow adjustment by everyone. In addition, survivors are helped to deal with the death. If the hospice care is at home, clients are in familiar surroundings, have their favorite food, and are close to loved ones.

The hospice does have disadvantages. One problem is whether family members, with a hospice's help, can handle the care at home. It may be too much, physically and emotionally. Also, what about dying clients? Are they comfortable with the kind of care they receive in the hospice? Do they need or want more? Are they comfortable in dealing with death? We may be conditioned to expect dying clients to be in hospitals, not homes. One research study indicated that 80 percent of relatives preferred to have their terminally ill loved ones die in the hospital, whereas 80 percent of dying clients said they preferred to die at home.[2]

Vignette 13

When executing a living will of a 76-year-old man who has been advised to have kidney dialysis, whose authority is paramount when there is disagreement among the nephrologist, the primary care physician, the client, and the family?

Later the same client is on the dialysis machine, and wants to discontinue the machine against the advice of the nephrologist. Has the authority changed?

Would the authority change in either of the two preceding situations if dialysis is performed while the client is a hospital inpatient as opposed to a client in a dialysis center?

ASSISTED SUICIDE

Questions arise about whether physician-assisted suicide or euthanasia should be endorsed. Are the two similar, or are they different enough that the arguments for one do not apply to the other? It is physician-assisted suicide when the physician gives a client a lethal dose of medication so that the client can self-administer the medication; it is active euthanasia when a physician administers a lethal dose to the client. In either case of physician-assisted suicide or euthanasia, the physician is active and involved; however, in both cases the client decides whether to ask for the medication. The client makes the choices in dying. In physician-assisted suicide, the client acts last, whereas in active euthanasia, the physician acts last.[3]

Just as California and Washington were forerunners with their living wills and natural death laws, they were forerunners in seeking legislation that would give people the option to seek "aid in dying from physicians to end life in a dignified, painless and humane manner." Such proposed laws are much broader in their scope than any living will or physicians' directive. One example is Washington Initiative 119, which was defeated by the voters. This proposed law would in effect have legalized active euthanasia. The text of the initiative specifically stated that the legislation should not be "construed to condone, authorize, or approve mercy killing," and the proposed law did not obligate any physician or health care institution to comply with a client's request for aid in dying. The initiative did propose, however, that (1) physicians who provide aid in dying would be immune from prosecution for criminal or unprofessional conduct and (2) physicians or facilities that did not choose to comply with such a client request must make a "good faith effort" to transfer the client to a physician or to another facility that will carry out the "medical service."[4]

In 1994 Oregon became the third state, after Washington and California, to ask voters to pass an assisted-suicide measure. It passed, but was challenged by the courts. Then in 1997, the assisted suicide measure was reaffirmed by the Oregon voters. The measure is the nation's first to allow a physician to prescribe a lethal dose of medication when asked by a terminally ill client. The four safeguards for this measure are as follows: (1) The attending physician must truly convey informed consent, which must include all feasible opportunities such as pain management, hospice, and palliative care. (2) The attending physician diagnosis and prognosis must be confirmed by a consulting physician. The latter physician must verify that the client has made a voluntary and informed decision. (3) If either physician thinks the client might have depression that might impair judgment, a counseling session must be made. (4) The client making the request must do so both orally and in writing. The law details specific time lines and a waiting period for the client before receiving the lethal medication. The request must be witnessed by at least two people who can verify the client's capacity to make a decision and that the decision is voluntary. Obviously, the measure poses valid concerns, but it is a testimony to the growing desire to have increased legal protection for options in dying.

CRITICAL THINKING EXERCISE

The U.S. Supreme Court recently ruled on Washington State's and New York State's assisted suicide laws. The nation's newspapers revealed that one justice's wife died of cancer, another justice is a cancer survivor, and a third justice's spouse works with cancer clients. They rejected the notion that assisted suicide is a fundamental liberty.

To ensure a person's ultimate choice, one physician has designed a procedure to help persons take their own lives. In June 1990 Dr. Jack Kevorkian allegedly used his "suicide machine" to assist in the death of 54-year-old Janet Adkins. Adkins was diagnosed as having Alzheimer's, a degenerative disease of the brain. She chose to end her life before she became incapacitated. Dr. Kevorkian was later arrested and charged with murder. The charge, however, was dismissed by the judge as insupportable. After allegedly assisting in the suicides of other people, however, Dr. Kevorkian has again been arrested and charged with murder. He has been ordered to stand trial again. At the date of publication, no guilty verdict is given.

On April 17, 1997, the U.S. Senate passed a bill barring the federal government from financing physician-assisted suicide. The vote was 99 to 0. The same measure previously cleared the House of Representatives by a vote of 398 to 16. Medicare and medicaid are prohibited from funding physician-assisted suicide. In June 1997, all nine Supreme Court justices refused to accept the fact that assisted suicide was a fundamental liberty for the terminally ill. Instead, they reinstated two state (Washington and New York) bans on the practice.

Legislation on physician-assisted suicide will be controversial, contradictory, confusing, and as emotional as legalization of abortion has been in the United States. Some questions to ponder on the subject include the following: What constitutes a lethal medication? How accurate can the prediction of death within 6 months be? Will a working definition of "terminal" be relaxed? Can physicians recognize depression or the inability of a client to make such a choice? What if the prescription fails to kill and the result debilitates the client? What happens to the client who asks for a lethal medication but is unable to administer it? Is that person's right less than the person who is able to administer the dose?

■■■ UNIFORM ANATOMICAL GIFT ACT

The legal definition of death is particularly important in the area of organ transplants. Under the old definitions, a surgeon removing a vital organ from a body still breathing and pulsating could technically be guilty of homicide. Many states, however, have adopted legislation making such actions possible. All 50 states have some form of the Uniform Anatomical Gift Act. Persons 18 years or older and of sound mind may make a gift of all or any part of their body to the following persons for the following purposes:

1. To any hospital, surgeon, or physician for medical or dental education, research, advancement of medical or dental science, therapy, or transplantation
2. To any accredited medical or dental school, college, or university for education, research, advancement of medical or dental science, or therapy
3. To any organ bank or storage facility, for medical or dental education, research, advancement of medical or dental science, therapy, or transplantation
4. To any specified individual for therapy or transplantation needed by him or her

The gift may be made by a provision in a will or by signing, in the presence of two witnesses, a card. The card is generally carried with the person at all times.[5] The latter method is the best because the living will may not be readily available until it is too late for donation of organs or tissues. Donated organs may include heart, lung, kidney, pancreas, liver, and intestine; tissue includes eyes, skin, bone, heart valves, veins, and tendons.

It is illegal to sell body parts in this country; however, the practice is common in developing countries. There is no cost to the family of the donor. Generally, there is no cost for later cremation or burial of the body parts.

Persons may place conditions on their organ donation. If a relative opposes the donation, most physicians and hospitals would not insist on the transplant. Donors are carefully screened before their body parts are used. The physician and hospital may be found negligent, so they must have strict standards for donor screening. Refer to Appendix II for a sample of the Uniform Donor Card.

Ethical issues include the following: What method is used to determine death in your state, and is it identified in the Uniform Anatomical Gift Act? The act is vague and does not specify the definition of death. Is dead really dead? Cultural differences exist, as well as religious differences in organ and tissue donation. For example, the Hmoges immigrant from Southeast Asia may believe that organ donation prevents the person from